THE **ALKAINE** HEALTHY DIET FOR KIDS

100+ Recipes for Your Health, To Lose Weight Naturally and Bring Your Body Back to Balance

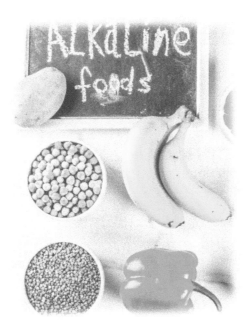

By

Laura Green

TABLE OF CONTENT

INTRODUCTION

Let's start with a bit of review of our chemistry lessons and remember what pH is. A simple definition is how much concentration of hydrogen ions there is in our body. The acronym pH is an abbreviation for "hydrogen potency." The "p" stands for "potent" or the German word for power, and "H" stands for the symbol for the element hydrogen. The pH scale ranges from 1 to 14. Seven is neutral. A pH below seven is acidic. Solutions that have a pH above seven are alkaline.

To have good health, our bodies must be somewhat alkaline. The pH of our blood and other cellular fluids should be around a pH between 7.365 and 7.45. It is essential to understand that pH levels vary significantly throughout the body. Some parts will be acidic, while others will be alkaline. There is no set level. For example, our stomach is loaded with hydrochloric acid, which gives it a pH of between 2 and 3.5. This makes it very acidic. It needs to be this acidic to break down the foods we consume and kill harmful bacteria. Our saliva has a pH between 6.8 and 7.3. Our skin has a pH between 4 and 6.5. This acts as a protective barrier from the environment. Our urine has a pH that ranges from alkaline to acidic. It all depends on what you eat.

The most critical measure is the pH of your blood. It needs to stay in a very narrow range between 7.365 and 7.45. This may sound simple, but instead of operating on a mathematical scale, our pH operates on a logarithmic scale in multiples of ten. This means that it will take ten times the amount of alkalinity to neutralize an acid. A pH of five will be 100 times more acidic than a pH of seven. A pH of four will be 1,000 times more acidic. Does this help you understand?

Don't start stressing about being in or out of this range. Remember that our bodies are pretty good at regulating the pH of our blood. However, our bodies do not "find" the balance. It has many parts that do, and it keeps the blood pH between 7.365 and 7.45 at all times. If you make poor lifestyle and food choices, your body works harder to maintain balance. If you want to address inflammation and acidity in your body by changing your food choices to more alkaline foods, this will help balance your system and bring your body back to its best vitality.

BLOOD pH

You know that the body is constantly working to maintain healthy pH levels in your body. The tricky thing is that three fluids in the body are typically at slightly different pH levels. But overall, they're primarily controlled by the same things. So the first thing we're going to look at is blood pH.

The normal pH range for blood is 7.35 to 7.45. This means that blood is usually alkaline or basic by nature. However, compared to stomach acid, which is between 3 and 5.5, a significant difference can be seen. The stomach is supposed to be at this acid level to break down the food you eat. Ironically, if your stomach acid becomes more acidic or more essential, it can create the same symptoms of acid reflux, but that's another matter. This low pH helps you digest your food and destroys germs that may enter your stomach.

What can cause your blood pH to change or reach abnormal levels?

Health problems are usually the most common cause of your blood becoming too alkaline or acidic. In addition, a change in normal blood pH levels can signal a medical emergency or health condition. This may include:

- Poisoning
- Drug overdose
- Bleeding
- Shock
- Infection
- Gout
- Lung disease

- Kidney disease
- Heart disease
- Diabetes
- Asthma

Acidosis refers to when the blood pH level drops below 7.35 and begins to become too acidic. Alkalosis refers to when the blood pH level rises to more than 7.45 and becomes too alkaline. Two main organs work hard to help maintain normal pH levels in the blood:

- Kidneys - These organs work by removing acid through urine to excrete it.
- Lungs - These organs work by getting rid of carbon dioxide through breathing.

The different forms of blood alkalosis and acidosis depend significantly on the cause. However, the two leading causes are:

- Metabolic - These types of problems occur most often when the pH of the blood changes due to a problem with a condition in the kidneys.
- Respiratory - These types of problems occur most often when the blood pH changes due to a respiratory or pulmonary condition.

It is common for blood pH levels to be tested as part of a blood gas test. This type of test is also called an ABG test or arterial blood gas test. It works by measuring how much carbon dioxide and oxygen are in your blood. Your primary care doctor may choose to test your blood pH as a regular part of your annual health screenings or if you already have certain health conditions. Blood pH testing requires drawing blood with a needle. The lab will receive the blood sample and perform the test.

There are blood pH tests you can do at home by pricking your finger. These tests will not give you an accurate reading like a test in your doctor's office. Using a urine pH test will not show you the pH level of your blood, but it can let you know if something is wrong.

Let's take a moment to take a closer look at some reasons why your blood pH levels are moving outside of the normal range.

High blood pH, also known as alkalosis, occurs if your blood pH rises above the normal range. There are many reasons for high blood pH levels. For example, you may have a temporary increase in blood pH with simple illnesses. Certain foods can also cause your blood to become more alkaline. However, there are also more serious causes for this alkalosis that can create additional problems.

The first is fluid loss. Losing too much water can cause the pH levels in your blood to rise. This is because you also lose certain electrolytes in your blood, minerals, and salts when you lose water. These include potassium and sodium. In addition, diarrhea, vomiting, and sweating can cause you to lose excess fluids.

Medications and diuretics can also cause a person to urinate more often, leading to increased pH levels in the blood. Treatment for fluid loss requires making sure to take plenty of fluids and replacing electrolytes. Some sports drinks can be used for this purpose. Your doctor can also review your medications and stop those that may be causing fluid loss.

Next, kidney problems can cause high pH levels in the blood. The kidneys play an essential role in maintaining normal blood pH. Therefore, a kidney problem can cause a buildup of alkalinity in the blood. This is because the kidneys do not remove excess alkaline substances through the urine. For example, the kidneys may improperly filter bicarbonate in the blood. Medications can regulate this.

When there is acidosis in the blood, it can affect the functioning of every organ in the body. Low blood pH is a more common problem than high blood pH. Therefore, acidosis is often a warning sign of some health problem that is not being controlled.

Some health conditions can cause natural acids to build up in the blood. Some forms of acids that can end up lowering the pH of the blood include:
- Carbonic acid
- Hydrochloric acid
- Phosphoric acid
- Sulfuric acid
- Ketogenic acids
- Lactic acid

An improper diet can cause problems. Eating an unbalanced diet can create a temporary low pH level in the blood. Not eating enough or going for long periods without eating can produce more acid in the blood. Try to avoid eating too many acid-forming foods, which include:
- Grains - rice, pasta, bread, and flour
- fish
- Meat
- Eggs
- Poultry - turkey and chicken
- Dairy products - yogurt, cheese, and cow's milk

Balance your blood pH by eating more alkaline foods. These include dried, frozen, and fresh fruits and fresh, cooked vegetables more often. Stay away from fad or starvation diets. Instead, when you're trying to lose weight, do so healthily and safely by following a balanced diet.

Another cause of low blood pH levels is due to diabetic ketoacidosis. If you have diabetes, your blood can end up turning acidic if you don't properly regulate your blood sugar levels. Diabetic ketoacidosis occurs when your body can't make enough insulin or use it properly.

Insulin helps move sugar from the foods we eat to the cells in the body. This is where the body burns it as fuel. If insulin cannot be used, the body begins to break down the fat stored in the body for energy. This releases a wasted acid known as ketones. If the body cannot regulate this process, the acid will build up and trigger a low pH in the blood.

You must seek emergency care if your blood sugar level exceeds 300 milligrams per deciliter. If you suffer from any of the following symptoms, talk to your doctor:
- Confusion
- Stomach pain
- Shortness of breath
- Shortness of breath
- Vomiting or nausea
- Weakness or fatigue
- Frequent urination
- Excessive thirst

Diabetic ketoacidosis is most often a sign that diabetes is not being treated properly and is out of control. This can sometimes be the first sign of diabetes for some people. Making sure your diabetes is well treated will help keep your blood pH in balance. It may require a strict diet and exercise plan, insulin injections, and medications to stay healthy.

The third cause of low blood pH is metabolic acidosis. This is when low blood pH is caused by kidney disease or failure. This occurs when there is a kidneys failure to remove acids from the body through urination. This will increase the acids in the body and lower the pH of the blood.

The most common symptoms of metabolic acidosis include

- Heavy breathing
- Fast heartbeat
- Headaches
- Vomiting and nausea
- Loss of appetite
- Weakness and fatigue

Treatment for this problem often includes medications to help the kidneys work better, but a kidney transplant or dialysis is the only solution for severe cases. Dialysis works by cleansing the blood.

The final cause of low pH in the blood is respiratory acidosis. When the lungs are probably not working to remove carbon dioxide from the body quickly, blood pH levels drop. This will happen more often if a person has a chronic or severe lung condition, such as:

- Diaphragm disorders
- Chronic obstructive pulmonary disease
- Pneumonia
- Bronchitis
- Sleep apnea
- Asthma

People who are obese, have had surgery, or abuse opioid painkillers or sedatives are at increased risk of developing respiratory acidosis. In some cases, the kidneys can take over and remove excess blood acids through excretion. As a result, a person may need to receive extra oxygen and medications such as steroids and bronchodilators to help the lungs function correctly. In very severe cases, mechanical ventilation and intubation may be necessary for individuals with respiratory acidosis to bring the blood pH back to normal.

- Urine pH

The next type of pH we will examine is that of urine. Urine is composed of waste products, salts, and water that are excreted through the kidneys. The balance of these different compounds can affect the acidity level of the urine. According to the American Association for Clinical Chemistry, the average urine pH is 6.0, but it can range from 4.5 to 8.0. Any level below 5.0 is considered acidic urine, and any level above 8.0 is considered primary urine.

Sometimes different labs have different ranges on what they consider normal pH levels for urine. One of the main things that affect the pH of your urine is the things you eat. If you go to your doctor, he or she will often ask you what foods you ate before evaluating the results of a urine pH test.

If, before a test, you ate more acidic foods, your urine will be more acidic. The same is true if you have eaten more alkaline foods. If a person has extremely high pH levels in their urine, meaning it is more alkaline, it could be the result of problems such as

- Urinary tract infections
- Kidney stones
- Other kidney-related disorders

A person may also have high pH levels in their urine if they have had prolonged vomiting. This is because vomiting causes the body to get rid of stomach acid, which causes the body's fluids to become more essential.

When urine is acidic, it creates an environment conducive to kidney stones. When urine is acidic, it can also be a sign of several severe medical conditions, such as:

- Hunger
- Diarrhea
- Diabetic ketoacidosis

As you'll notice, much of this is the same as blood pH levels. Some medications can affect the pH of the urine. Sometimes doctors will ask the patient to discontinue certain medications the day or night before doing a urinalysis.

- Saliva pH

The final pH we will look at is the pH of saliva. The usual range of saliva pH is 6.2 to 7.6. The things you drink and eat can change the pH of your saliva.

Just like any other area of your body, your mouth needs to maintain a balanced pH. Saliva pH levels can drop below 5.5 when you've had a lot of acidic drinks. In this case, the acids in your mouth begin to break down the enamel on your teeth.

If the enamel on your teeth becomes too thin, the dentin will be exposed. This can end up causing discomfort when you consume sugary, cold, or hot drinks. Just to give you an example of foods and drinks that can do this, here are some numbers:

- Cherries have a pH of 4
- American cheese has a pH of 5
- White wine has a pH of 4
- Soft drinks have a pH of 3

It's easy to spot unbalanced pH levels in your saliva. Some of the most common indicators are:

- Tooth decay
- Sensitivity to cold or hot drinks or foods
- Persistent bad breath

If you want, you can also test the pH of your saliva. The pH of your saliva can be tested: you'll need to find pH strips. Once you have the strips, here's what you need to do:

- Make sure you don't eat or drink anything for at least two hours before the test.
- Let your mouth fill with saliva and then swallow or spit it out.
- Let your mouth fill with saliva again, and then put a small amount on one of your pH strips.
- The strip will then react to your saliva. It will change color based on how alkaline or acidic your saliva is. The container the pH strips came with should show a color chart. Place your strip next to the chart to match the colors and determine the pH level of your saliva.

To make sure the pH of your saliva stays balanced, you need to eat foods that are in a healthy pH range. It is also to continue absorb essential vitamins and minerals. There are some more effective ways to make sure the pH of your saliva stays balanced.

- Stay away from sugary drinks. If you must drink them, try to swig them and chase them with water. Sipping sugary beverages for an extended period does more damage.
- Limit black coffee. Adding a little cream, unsweetened, can help reduce the acidity of coffee.
- Avoid brushing your teeth immediately after consuming high-acid beverages such as beer, wine, cider, juice, or soda. These types of beverages soften tooth enamel.
- Chew sugar-free gum after consuming any beverage or food. Chewing gum causes your mouth to produce more saliva and helps bring your pH level back to normal. It is also believed that xylitol can prevent bacteria from sticking to your tooth enamel. Always remember to keep yourself hydrated, so be sure to drink plenty of water.

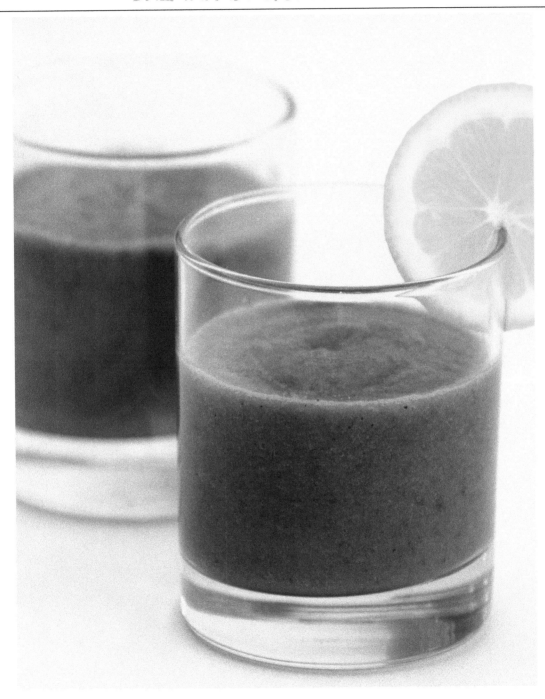

1) Baked walnut oatmeal

Preparation time: 15 minutes

Cooking time: 45 minutes

Portions: 5

Ingredients:

- ✓ 1 tablespoon linseed meal
- ✓ 3 tablespoons of alkaline water
- ✓ 3 cups unsweetened almond milk
- ✓ ¼ cup maple syrup
- ✓ 2 tablespoons coconut oil, melted and cooled
- ✓ 2 teaspoons of organic vanilla extract

Ingredients:

- ✓ 1 teaspoon cinnamon powder
- ✓ 1 teaspoon organic baking powder
- ✓ ¼ teaspoon of sea salt
- ✓ 2 cups old rolled oats
- ✓ ½ cup almonds, chopped
- ✓ ½ cup walnuts, chopped

Directions:

- ❖ Lightly grease an 8x8-inch baking dish. Set aside.
- ❖ In a large bowl, add the flaxseed meal and water and beat until well combined. Set aside for about 5 minutes.
- ❖ In the bowl of the flax mixture, add the remaining ingredients except the oats and nuts and mix until well combined.
- ❖ Add the oats and nuts and stir gently to combine.
- ❖ Place the mixture in the prepared baking tin and spread it out in an even layer.
- ❖ Cover the baking tray with plastic wrap and refrigerate for about 8 hours.
- ❖ Preheat the oven to 350 degrees F. Place a wire rack in the centre of the oven.
- ❖ Remove the tray from the refrigerator and let it rest at room temperature for 15-20 minutes.
- ❖ Remove the plastic film and mix the oatmeal mixture well.
- ❖ Bake for about 45 minutes.
- ❖ Remove from the oven and set aside to cool slightly.
- ❖ Serve hot.

2) Banana waffles

Preparation time: 15 minutes

Cooking time: 20 minutes

Portions: 5

Ingredients:

- ✓ 2 tablespoons of linseed flour
- ✓ 6 tablespoons of warm alkaline water
- ✓ 2 bananas, peeled and mashed

Ingredients:

- ✓ 1 cup creamy almond butter
- ✓ ¼ cup whole coconut milk

Directions:

- ❖ In a small bowl, add the linseed flour and warm water and whisk until well combined.
- ❖ Set aside for about 10 minutes or until the mixture becomes thick.
- ❖ In a medium bowl, add the bananas, almond butter and coconut milk, mix well.
- ❖ Add the flax meal mixture and stir until well combined.
- ❖ Preheat the waffle iron and grease it lightly.
- ❖ Place the desired amount of batter in the preheated waffle iron.
- ❖ Cook for about 3-4 minutes or until the wafers turn golden brown.
- ❖ Repeat with the remaining mixture.
- ❖ Serve hot.

3) Savoury sweet potato waffles

Preparation time: 10 minutes   **Cooking time:** 20 minutes   **Portions: 2**

Ingredients:

- ✓ 1 medium sweet potato, peeled, grated and squeezed
- ✓ 1 teaspoon fresh thyme, chopped
- ✓ 1 teaspoon fresh rosemary, chopped

Ingredients:

- ✓ 1/8 teaspoon red pepper flakes, crushed
- ✓ Sea salt and freshly ground black pepper, to taste

Directions:

- ❖ Preheat the waffle iron and then grease it.
- ❖ In a large bowl, add all the ingredients and mix until well combined.
- ❖ Put ½ of the sweet potato mixture into the preheated waffle iron and bake for about 8-10 minutes or until golden brown.
- ❖ Repeat with the remaining mixture.
- ❖ Serve hot.

4) Oatmeal and fruit pancakes

Preparation time: 10 minutes   **Cooking time:** 15 minutes   **Portions: 3**

Ingredients:

- ✓ 1 cup rolled oats
- ✓ 1 medium banana, peeled and mashed
- ✓ ¼-½ cup unsweetened almond milk
- ✓ 1 tablespoon organic baking powder

Ingredients:

- ✓ 1 tablespoon organic apple cider vinegar
- ✓ 1 tablespoon agave nectar
- ✓ ½ teaspoon organic vanilla extract
- ✓ ½ cup of fresh blackberries

Directions:

- ❖ Place all the ingredients except the blackberries in a large bowl and mix until well combined.
- ❖ Gently add the blackberries.
- ❖ Set the mixture aside for about 5-10 minutes.
- ❖ Preheat a large non-stick frying pan over medium-low heat.
- ❖ Add about ¼ cup of the mixture and with a spatula, spread into an even layer.
- ❖ Immediately, cover the pan and cook for about 2-3 minutes or until golden brown.
- ❖ Flip the pancake over and bake for a further 1-2 minutes or until golden brown.
- ❖ Repeat with the remaining mixture.
- ❖ Serve hot.

5) Frozen banana breakfast bowl

Preparation time: **Cooking time:**   **Portions: 1**

Ingredients:

- ✓ Chia seeds, hemp seeds, unsweetened coconut flakes, for garnish - optional
- ✓ Pumpkin seed protein powder, 4 tablespoons

Ingredients:

- ✓ Bananas, 2

Directions:

- ❖ Peel and then slice the bananas. Place them thinly in a freezer-safe container and freeze overnight.
- ❖ The next morning, add the bananas to a food processor and blend until a smooth, creamy consistency is achieved, much like that of soft-serve ice cream.
- ❖ Process the pumpkin protein powder through the bananas until it is just combined.
- ❖ Pour into a serving dish and add the desired toppings, if desired, and enjoy.

6) Chia seed and blueberry cobbler

Preparation time: **Cooking time:**   **Portions: 4**

Ingredients:

- ✓ Blueberry mixture -
- ✓ Chia seeds, 1 tablespoon
- ✓ Unrefined whole cane sugar, 2 tablespoons
- ✓ Blueberries, 2 c.
- ✓ Topping -
- ✓ Almond flour, .5 c.
- ✓ Sea salt, .25 teaspoon
- ✓ Vanilla pod powder, 1 teaspoon

Ingredients:

- ✓ A mixture of bicarbonate of soda and cream of tartar, 1.5 teaspoons
- ✓ Unrefined whole cane sugar, 2 tablespoons
- ✓ Melted coconut oil, 2 tablespoons
- ✓ Coconut milk, 4 tablespoons
- ✓ Oatmeal, .5 c.

Directions:

- ❖ Start by setting your oven to 350.
- ❖ To make the blueberries, mix the chia seeds, sugar and blueberries. Place the blueberry mixture in the bottom of four 4-ounce baking cups.
- ❖ To make the topping, mix together the salt, vanilla powder, baking powder, sugar, coconut oil, coconut milk, oatmeal and almond flour.

- ❖ Divide the blueberry topping between the four ramekins. You can leave the topping by spoonfuls, or you can spread it evenly over the blueberry mixture to create a complete crust.
- ❖ Bake the cobblers for 45 minutes, or until the topping has turned golden brown and everything is heated through. Enjoy.

7) Quick and easy granola bars

Preparation time:

Cooking time:

Portions: 6

Ingredients:

- ✓ Vanilla pod powder, .25 teaspoon
- ✓ Cinnamon spice, .25 teaspoon
- ✓ Sea salt, .25 teaspoon
- ✓ Coconut oil, 1 tablespoon

Ingredients:

- ✓ Brown rice syrup, 2 tablespoons
- ✓ Almond butter, .5 c.
- ✓ Rolled quick oats, 1 c.

Directions:

- ❖ Place some parchment in the bottom of a 9x5 inch baking tin.
- ❖ Add the vanilla pod powder, cinnamon, salt, coconut oil, brown rice syrup, almond butter and oats to a food processor and blend until well combined.

- ❖ Slide the dough into the baking tray and press it down into an even dough, making sure it is well compressed. Refrigerate the bars for 15-20 minutes, or until they are completely firm.
- ❖ Cut the granola into six bars and enjoy. Store the leftovers in the fridge. At room temperature, they will become soft.

8) Alkaline Blueberry Spelt Pancakes

Preparation time: 6 mnutes.

Cooking time: 20 minutes.

Portions: 3

Ingredients:

- ✓ 2 cups of spelt flour
- ✓ 1 cup coconut Milk
- ✓ 1/2 cup Alkaline Water
- ✓ 2 tbsps. Grape sed Oil

Ingredients:

- ✓ 1/2 cup Agave
- ✓ 1/2 cup Blueberries
- ✓ 1/4 teaspoon musk Sea

Directions:

- ❖ Mix together in a whisk the spellated flower, agave, wheat sed oil, hemp seeds and moss5s together.
- ❖ To the menstruum, add 1 cup of sheep's milk and cologne until you get the consistency menstruum you like.

- ❖ Mash the blue into the batter.
- ❖ Heat over medium heat and then lightly coat with the cereal oil.
- ❖ Put the butter in the oven and let it cook for about 5 minutes on all sides.
- ❖ Serve and have fun.

9) Alkaline blueberry muffins

Preparation time: 5 Minutes.

Cooking time: 20 minutes.

Portions: 3

Ingredients:

- ✓ 1 cup of coconut milk
- ✓ 3/4 cup of Spelt Flour
- ✓ 3/4 Teff flour
- ✓ 1/2 cup Blueberries

Ingredients:

- ✓ 1/3 cup of Agave
- ✓ 1/4 cup Sea Moss Gel
- ✓ 1/2 teaspoon coarse salt, ground salt, olive oil

Directions:

- ❖ Adjust the oven temperature to 365 degrees.
- ❖ Grate 6 regular-size muffin cups with muffin liners.
- ❖ In a bowl, mix the sea salt, moss, agave, nut milk and flour until liquid.

- ❖ Then crimp in blueberries.
- ❖ Cover the muffins lightly with the wheat seeds.
- ❖ Pour in the batter of muffin.
- ❖ Bake for at least 30 minutes until golden brown.
- ❖ Serve.

10) Meal of crispy quinoa

Preparation time: 5 minutes

Cooking time: 25 minutes.

Portions: 2

Ingredients:
- ✓ 3 cups of nut milk coco
- ✓ 1 cup rinsed quinoa.
- ✓ 1/8 tsp. cinnamon powder

Directions:
- ❖ In a saucepan, your milk and bring to a boil over moderate heat.
- ❖ Add the milk and then soak it once more.
- ❖ Then leave to stand for at least 15 minutes over a medium heat until the milk has reduced.

Ingredients:
- ✓ 1 cup raspberry
- ✓ 1/2 coconut

- ❖ Being higher in the corner than in the middle of the world.
- ❖ Cook for 8 minutes until the milk is ready to use.
- ❖ Add the raspberry and coook the meal for 30 seconds.
- ❖ Serve enjoy.

11) Coconut pancakes

Preparation time: 5 minutes.

Cooking time: 15 minutes.

Portions: 4

Ingredients:
- ✓ 1 cup coconut flour
- ✓ 2 tbsps. Arrow root powder
- ✓ 1 tsp. baking powder

Directions:
- ❖ In a medium container, mix all the ingredients.
- ❖ Add the coconut milk and 2 tbsps. Del coconut oil and mix properly.
- ❖ In a frying pan, melt 1 tsp. of coco walnut oil.
- ❖ Pour a ladleful of batter into the container and then spread the batter evenly on a smooth surface.

Ingredients:
- ✓ 1 cup coco walnut milk
- ✓ 3 tbsps. Coconut oil

- ❖ Coook il form for a least 3 minutes on average heat until you becomes firm.
- ❖ Flip the pancake onto the other side and cook for a further 2 minutes until golden brown.
- ❖ Cook the pancakes in a microwave oven.
- ❖ Serve.

12) Quinoa Porridge

Preparation time: 5 minutes.

Cooking time: 25 minutes.

Portions: 2

Ingredients:
- ✓ 2 cups coco nut milk
- ✓ 1 cup rinsed quinoa.

Directions:
- ❖ In a saucepan, boil the nut milk at a high temperature.
- ❖ Add the quinoa to the milk and then bring the mixture to a boil.
- ❖ Then you let it sit for 15 mnutes on medium heat until the milk has reduced.

Ingredients:
- ✓ 1/8 tsp. ground cinnamon
- ✓ 1 cup fresh blueberries

- ❖ Add the cinnamon and then mix well in the fridge.
- ❖ Cook for at least 8 minutes until the milk is absorbed.
- ❖ Add the blue and light blue and then mix for a further 30 seconds.
- ❖ Serve.

13) Amaranth porridge

Preparation time: 5 minutes.

Cooking time: 30 minutes.

Portions: 2

Ingredients:
- ✓ 2 cups coconut milk
- ✓ 2 cups alkaline water
- ✓ 1 cup of administrator

Directions:
- ❖ In a bowl, mix the milk with the water and then boil the milk.

Ingredients:
- ✓ 2 tbsps. Coconut oil
- ✓ 1 tbsp. land cinnamon

- ❖ You put in the amaranth and then reduce the heat and make milk.

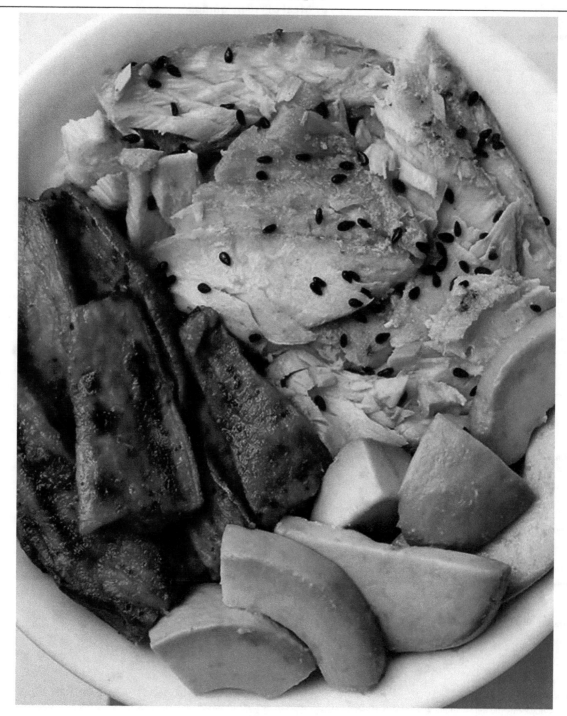

14) Wakame and pepper salad

Preparation time: 15 minutes   **Cooking time**: 0 minutes   **Portions: 2**

Ingredients:
- ✓ 1 cup of wakame stalks
- ✓ ½ tablespoon chopped red pepper
- ✓ ½ teaspoon of onion powder
- ✓ ½ tablespoon lime juice

Directions:
- ❖ Put the wakame stalks in a bowl, cover with water, let them soak for 10 minutes and then drain.
- ❖ Meanwhile, prepare the dressing and for this, take a small bowl, add the lime juice, onion, agave syrup and sesame oil and then whisk until combined.

Ingredients:
- ✓ ½ tablespoon agave syrup
- ✓ ½ tablespoon sesame seeds
- ✓ ½ tablespoon sesame oil

- ❖ Place the drained wakame stalks in a large dish, add the pepper, pour in the seasoning and stir until coated.
- ❖ Sprinkle the salad with sesame seeds and serve.

15) Green salad of orange and avocado

Preparation time: 5 minutes   **Cooking time:** 0 minutes   **Portions: 2**

Ingredients:
- ✓ 1 orange, peeled, sliced
- ✓ 4 cups of vegetables
- ✓ ½ avocado, peeled, pitted and diced
- ✓ 2 tablespoons chopped red onion
- ✓ ½ cup of coriander

Directions:
- ❖ Prepare the dressing and for this, place the coriander in a food processor, pour in the orange juice, lime juice and oil, add the salt and then pulse until combined.

Ingredients:
- ✓ ¼ teaspoon of salt
- ✓ ¼ cup of olive oil
- ✓ 2 tablespoons of lime juice
- ✓ 2 tablespoons of orange juice

- ❖ Pour the dressing into a jar. Add the remaining ingredients, stir until coated and add to a salad bowl or serve in the jar.

16) Green salad with cucumbers and mushrooms

Preparation time: 5 minutes   **Cooking time:** 0 minutes   **Portions: 2**

Ingredients:
- ✓ ½ medium-sized cucumber, seedless, chopped
- ✓ 6 lettuce leaves, broken into pieces
- ✓ 4 mushrooms, chopped
- ✓ 6 cherry tomatoes, chopped

Directions:
- ❖ Take a medium salad bowl, put all the ingredients in it and then toss until mixed.

Ingredients:
- ✓ 10 olives
- ✓ ½ of a lime, squeezed
- ✓ 1 teaspoon of olive oil
- ✓ ¼ teaspoon of salt
- ❖ Serve immediately.

17) Chickpea, vegetable and fonio salad

Preparation time: 10 minutes   **Cooking time:** 5 minutes   **Portions: 2**

Ingredients:
- ✓ ½ cup of cooked chickpeas
- ✓ ¼ cup chopped cucumber
- ✓ ½ cup crushed red pepper
- ✓ ½ cup cherry tomatoes, halved
- ✓ ½ cup of fonio

Directions:
- ❖ Take a medium saucepan, place it over high heat, pour in the water and bring it to the boil.
- ❖ Add the fonio, lower the heat, cook for 1 minute and then remove the pan from the heat.

Ingredients:
- ✓ ⅓ teaspoon of salt
- ✓ 1 tablespoon of grape oil
- ✓ ⅛ teaspoon of cayenne pepper
- ✓ 1 key file, squeezed
- ✓ 1 cup of spring water
- ❖ Cover the pot with its lid, let the fonio stand for 5 minutes, mash it with a fork and then leave it to cool for 15 minutes.
- ❖ Take a salad bowl, put in the lime juice and oil and then stir in the salt and cayenne pepper until combined.
- ❖ Add the remaining ingredients, including the fonio, stir until combined, then serve.

18) Avocado and chickpea salad

Preparation time: 10 minutes   **Cooking time**: 20 minutes   **Portions**: 2

Ingredients:
- ✓ ½ cucumber, seedless, sliced
- ✓ 2 avocados, peeled, pitted and diced
- ✓ 1 medium white onion, peeled, diced
- ✓ 2 cups of cooked chickpeas
- ✓ ¼ cup chopped coriander
- ✓ 1 teaspoon of onion powder

Ingredients:
- ✓ ½ teaspoon of cayenne pepper
- ✓ 1 teaspoon sea salt
- ✓ 2 tablespoons hemp seeds, shelled
- ✓ 1 key file, squeezed
- ✓ 1 tablespoon olive oil

Directions:
- ❖ Turn on the oven, then set it to 425ºF (220ºC) and let it preheat.
- ❖ Meanwhile, take a baking tray, place the chickpeas on it, season with salt, onion powder and pepper, drizzle with oil and then toss until combined.

- ❖ Cook the chickpeas for 20 minutes or until golden and crispy, then leave to cool for 10 minutes.
- ❖ Transfer the chickpeas to a bowl, add the remaining ingredients and stir until combined. Serve immediately.

19) Amaranth, cucumber and chickpea salad

Preparation time: 5 minutes   **Cooking time**: 10 minutes   **Portions**: 2

Ingredients:
- ✓ 1 small white onion, peeled, chopped
- ✓ 1 cup cooked amaranth
- ✓ ½ cucumber, seedless, chopped
- ✓ 1 cup of cooked chickpeas

Ingredients:
- ✓ ½ of a medium red pepper, chopped
- ✓ ⅓ teaspoon of sea salt
- ✓ ⅛ teaspoon of cayenne pepper
- ✓ 2 tablespoons of lime juice
- ❖ Place the remaining ingredients in a salad bowl, drizzle with the lime juice mixture, mix and serve.

Directions:
- ❖ Take a small bowl, put in the lime juice, add salt and stir until combined.

20) Avocado and rocket salad with citrus fruits

Preparation time: 5 minutes   **Cooking time:** 0 minutes   **Portions: 2**

Ingredients:
- ✓ 4 slices of onion
- ✓ ½ avocado, peeled, pitted and sliced
- ✓ 4 ounces (113 g) arugula
- ✓ 1 orange, peeled and sliced
- ✓ 1 teaspoon agave syrup

Directions:
- ❖ Distribute avocado, oranges, onion and rocket between two plates.

Ingredients:
- ✓ ⅛ teaspoon of salt
- ✓ ⅛ teaspoon of cayenne pepper
- ✓ 2 tablespoons of lime juice
- ✓ 2 tablespoons of olive oil

- ❖ Mix together the oil, salt, cayenne pepper, agave syrup and lime juice in a small bowl and then stir until combined.
- ❖ Pour the dressing over the salad and then serve.

21) Avocado salad and spelt noodles

Preparation time: 10 minutes   **Cooking time:** 0 minutes   **Portions: 2**

Ingredients:
- ✓ ½ cup avocado, peeled, pitted and chopped
- ✓ ½ cup of basil leaves
- ✓ ½ cup cherry tomatoes
- ✓ 2 cups of cooked spelt noodles

Directions:
- ❖ Take a large bowl, put the pasta in it, add the tomato, avocado and basil and then mix until everything is combined.
- ❖ Take a small bowl, add the agave syrup and salt, pour in the lime juice and olive oil, and then whisk until combined.

388 | fat: 16.5g | protein: 9.3g | carbohydrate: 54.2g | fibre: 8.5g

Ingredients:
- ✓ 1 teaspoon agave syrup
- ✓ 1 tablespoon lime juice
- ✓ 2 tablespoons of olive oil

- ❖ Pour the lime juice mixture over the pasta, stir until combined and then serve.

22) Lettuce salad with basil

Preparation time: 10 minutes   **Cooking time:** 10 minutes   **Portions: 2**

Ingredients:
- ✓ 2 small heads of romaine lettuce, cut in half
- ✓ 1 tablespoon chopped basil
- ✓ 1 tablespoon chopped red onion
- ✓ ¼ teaspoon of onion powder
- ✓ ½ tablespoon agave syrup

Directions:
- ❖ Take a large frying pan, put it over a medium heat and when it is hot, place the heads of lettuce in it, cut side down, and then cook them for 4 to 5 minutes per side until they are golden brown on both sides.
- ❖ When finished, transfer the heads of lettuce to a plate and leave to cool for 5 minutes.

Ingredients:
- ✓ ½ teaspoon of salt
- ✓ ¼ teaspoon cayenne pepper
- ✓ 2 tablespoons of olive oil
- ✓ 1 tablespoon lime juice

- ❖ In the meantime, prepare the dressing and for this, place the remaining ingredients in a small bowl and then mix until combined.
- ❖ Pour the dressing over the heads of lettuce and then serve.

23) Cabbage and sprout salad

Preparation time: 5 minutes   **Cooking time:** 0 minutes   **Portions: 2**

Ingredients:
- ✓ 2 cups of kale leaves
- ✓ 1 cup of sprouts
- ✓ 1 cup cherry tomatoes
- ✓ ½ avocado, peeled, pitted and diced

Directions:
- ❖ Take a small bowl, put the lime juice in it, add the oil and agave syrup and then stir until combined.

Ingredients:
- ✓ 1 key file, squeezed
- ✓ 1 teaspoon agave syrup
- ✓ ½ tablespoon olive oil
- ✓ ⅛ teaspoon of cayenne pepper

- ❖ Take a salad bowl, put the remaining ingredients in, drizzle with the lime juice mixture and then toss until mixed.
- ❖ Serve immediately.

24) Watercress and cucumber salad

Preparation time: 5 minutes   **Cooking time**: 0 minutes   **Portions: 2**

Ingredients:
- ✓ 2 cups of torn cress
- ✓ ½ sliced cucumber
- ✓ 1 tablespoon lime juice

Directions:
- ❖ Pour the lime juice and olive oil into a salad bowl and mix well to combine.
- ❖ Slice the cucumber and add it to the bowl.

Ingredients:
- ✓ 2 tablespoons of olive oil
- ✓ Pure sea salt, to taste
- ✓ Cayenne powder, to taste
- ❖ Tear up the watercress and add it to the bowl.
- ❖ Sprinkle with cayenne powder and pure sea salt according to your taste.
- ❖ Mix thoroughly.
- ❖ Serve immediately.

25) Watercress and orange salad

Preparation time: 10 minutes   **Cooking time**: 0 minutes   **Portions: 2**

Ingredients:
- ✓ 4 cups of torn cress
- ✓ 1 sliced avocado
- ✓ 2 thinly sliced red onions
- ✓ 1 Seville orange, chopped
- ✓ 2 tablespoons of lime juice

Directions:
- ❖ Prepare the avocado. cut it in half, peel it, remove the seeds and slice it.
- ❖ Peel the Seville orange and cut it into medium cubes.
- ❖ Remove the skin from the red onions and slice them thinly.

Ingredients:
- ✓ 2 teaspoons agave syrup
- ✓ ⅛ teaspoon of pure sea salt
- ✓ Cayenne powder, to taste
- ✓ 2 tablespoons of olive oil

- ❖ Put the onions, avocado, oranges and watercress in a salad bowl.
- ❖ Combine the olive oil, cayenne powder, pure sea salt, lime juice and agave syrup in a separate bowl, mix well.
- ❖ Pour the dressing over the top of the salad.
- ❖ Serve immediately.

26) Mushroom and olive salad

Preparation time: 10 minutes   **Cooking time**: 0 minutes   **Portions: 2**

Ingredients:
- ✓ 5 mushrooms cut in half
- ✓ 6 halved cherry (plum) tomatoes
- ✓ 6 lettuce leaves, rinsed
- ✓ 10 olives

Directions:
- ❖ Cut the rinsed lettuce leaves into medium pieces and place them in a medium salad bowl.
- ❖ Add the mushroom halves, chopped cucumber, olives and cherry tomato halves to the bowl.

Ingredients:
- ✓ ½ chopped cucumber
- ✓ Juice of ½ lime
- ✓ 1 teaspoon of olive oil
- ✓ Pure sea salt, to taste
- ❖ Stir well.
- ❖ Pour olive oil and lime juice over the salad.
- ❖ Add pure sea salt to taste. stir until well combined.
- ❖ Serve immediately.

27) Asparagus salad with cashew sauce

Preparation time: 10 minutes   **Cooking time**: 5 minutes   **Portions**: 1-2

Ingredients:

For the salad:
- ✓ 1 teaspoon avocado oil
- ✓ 24 asparagus stalks, diced
- ✓ ½ cup diced onion
- ✓ 3 cloves of garlic, crushed
- ✓ ½ teaspoon of sea salt
- ✓ ¼ teaspoon freshly ground black pepper

Directions:

- ❖ To prepare the asparagus mixture
- ❖ In a large frying pan over medium heat, heat the avocado oil. Add the asparagus, onion, garlic, salt and pepper and fry for 5-7 minutes, or until the onion is soft.

Ingredients:

For the dressing:
- ✓ ½ cup of raw cashews
- ✓ ½ cup of water
- ✓ 2 tablespoons freshly squeezed lemon juice
- ✓ ¼ teaspoon of sea salt
- ✓ ⅛ teaspoon of freshly ground black pepper
  For mounting:
- ✓ 2 cups of mixed salad
- ✓ To prepare the asparagus mixture
- ❖ Prepare the dressing
- ❖ In a high-speed blender, blend together half of the asparagus mixture with the cashews, water, lemon juice, salt and pepper until smooth.
- ❖ To assemble the salad
- ❖ Arrange the salad mix on 1 large or 2 small plates. Add the rest of the asparagus, drizzle with the dressing and enjoy.

28) Sweet potato salad with jalapeno sauce

Preparation time: 10 minutes   **Cooking time**: 25 minutes   **Portions**: 1-2

Ingredients:

For sweet potatoes:
- ✓ 3 medium sweet potatoes, peeled and diced
- ✓ 2 tablespoons of avocado oil
- ✓ 2 cloves of garlic, crushed
- ✓ 1 teaspoon ground paprika
- ✓ ½ teaspoon of sea salt
- ✓ For Jalapeño Dressing:
- ✓ 1 cup of water
- ✓ 1 cup raw cashews

Directions:

- ❖ Preheat the oven to 350°F (180°C). Line a baking tray with baking paper.
- ❖ To prepare the sweet potatoes
- ❖ In a medium bowl, mix the sweet potatoes, avocado oil, garlic, paprika and salt.
- ❖ Spread the sweet potato cubes evenly over the prepared baking tray and bake for 25 minutes, or until soft.

Ingredients:

- ✓ ¼ cup of fresh coriander leaves
- ✓ ½ to 1 jalapeño
- ✓ 2 tablespoons freshly squeezed lime juice
- ✓ ½ teaspoon of sea salt
  For mounting:
- ✓ 2 cups of mixed salad

- ❖ To prepare the jalapeño dressing
- ❖ Meanwhile, in a high-speed blender, blend together the water, cashews, cilantro, jalapeño, lime juice and salt until smooth.
- ❖ To assemble
- ❖ Arrange the salad mix on 1 large or 2 small plates. Add the hot sweet potatoes, drizzle with the dressing and enjoy.

29) Green pineapple salad

Preparation time: 10 minutes   **Cooking time**: 0 minutes   **Portions**: 1-2

Ingredients:

- ✓ For the lime vinaigrette:
- ✓ ¼ cup avocado oil
- ✓ ¼ cup of water
- ✓ 2 tablespoons freshly squeezed lime juice
- ✓ ½ cup chopped shallots
- ✓ ½ cup of chopped fresh coriander
- ✓ 2 garlic cloves
- ✓ ½ teaspoon of sea salt

Directions:

- ❖ To prepare the vinaigrette
- ❖ In a blender, blend together the avocado oil, water, lime juice, onion, cilantro, garlic and salt until well combined. Adjust the seasonings as necessary.

Ingredients:

- ✓ For mounting:
- ✓ 2 to 3 cups of mixed salad
- ✓ ½ cup of diced pineapple
- ✓ 1 cup chopped purple cabbage
- ✓ Dulse flakes, for garnish (optional)

- ❖ To assemble the salad
- ❖ Arrange the salad mix on 1 large or 2 small plates. Add the pineapple, purple cabbage and dulse flakes (if using); drizzle with the dressing and serve.

30) Sweet Peach Tahini Salad

Preparation time: 10 minutes   **Cooking time**: 0 minutes   **Portions**: 1-2

Ingredients:

- ✓ 4 tablespoons of tahini
- ✓ 3 to 4 tablespoons brown rice syrup
- ✓ ¼ cup of water
- ✓ 1 teaspoon freshly squeezed lemon juice
- ✓ Pinch of sea salt
- ✓ 1 peach, pitted and cut into cubes

Directions:

- ❖ In a small bowl, whisk together the tahini, brown rice syrup, water, lemon juice and salt until well combined. Adjust seasonings as needed.

Ingredients:

- ✓ ¼ cup diced red pepper
- ✓ 1 tablespoon fresh coriander, chopped
- ✓ 1 tablespoon diced red onion
- ✓ ½ jalapeño, diced
- ✓ 2 to 3 cups of mixed salad

- ❖ In another small bowl, put together the peach, pepper, cilantro, onion and jalapeño.
- ❖ Arrange the salad mix on 1 large or 2 small plates. Add the dressing, drizzle with the dressing and enjoy.

31) Pasta salad with red lentils and vegetables

Preparation time: 15 minutes   **Cooking time**: 15 minutes   **Portions**: 2-4

Ingredients:

- ✓ 2 cups of red lentil paste
- ✓ ¼ cup avocado oil
- ✓ 2 tablespoons apple cider vinegar
- ✓ 1 tablespoon freshly squeezed lemon juice
- ✓ 1 teaspoon dried oregano
- ✓ 2 pinches of sea salt
- ✓ 2 pinches of freshly ground black pepper

Directions:

- ❖ Cook the pasta according to the package directions.
- ❖ While the pasta is cooking, in a small bowl, whisk together the avocado oil, vinegar, lemon juice, oregano, salt and pepper until well combined. Adjust seasonings as needed.

Ingredients:

- ✓ 1 tablespoon avocado oil
- ✓ 6 asparagus stalks, diced
- ✓ 1 cup of diced orange pepper
- ✓ ⅓ cup of diced red onion
- ✓ ½ courgette, sliced
- ✓ ½ summer squash, sliced
- ✓ 2 cloves of garlic, crushed

- ❖ In a frying pan over medium-high heat, heat the avocado oil. Add the asparagus, pepper, onion, courgette, pumpkin and garlic and fry for 2 to 3 minutes, or just until soft.
- ❖ In a large bowl, mix the cooked pasta, vegetables and seasoning until well combined. Transfer to 2 large or 4 small plates and enjoy.

32) Fennel and carrot salad

Preparation time: 5 minutes   **Cooking time**: 0 minutes   **Portions**: 4

Ingredients:
- ✓ 1 cup chopped fennel
- ✓ 1 cup of shredded carrots
- ✓ ¼ cup sliced almonds
- ✓ 3 tablespoons of sultanas
- ✓ 1 tablespoon avocado oil

Ingredients:
- ✓ 1 tablespoon freshly squeezed lemon juice
- ✓ 1 teaspoon apple cider vinegar
- ✓ 1 teaspoon Dijon or yellow mustard
- ✓ 1 teaspoon of finely grated fresh ginger or 1 cube of frozen ginger

Directions:
- ❖ In a medium bowl, mix fennel, carrots, almonds and sultanas; set aside.
- ❖ In a small bowl, whisk together the oil, lemon juice, vinegar, mustard and ginger until well combined.
- ❖ Pour the dressing over the salad and toss until evenly coated.
- ❖ Serve cold or at room temperature. Store leftovers in an airtight container in the fridge for up to 1 week.

33) Tofu and watermelon salad

Preparation time: 10 minutes   **Cooking time**: 0 minutes   **Portions**: 4

Ingredients:
- ✓ 2 tablespoons freshly squeezed lemon juice
- ✓ 2 tablespoons of avocado oil
- ✓ 1 teaspoon dried oregano
- ✓ ½ teaspoon dried thyme
- ✓ ¼ teaspoon of garlic powder
- ✓ ¼ teaspoon of sea salt

Ingredients:
- ✓ 8 ounces (227 g) solid tofu, cubed
- ✓ ¼ cup balsamic vinegar
- ✓ 8 dates, pitted
- ✓ 4 cups of crunchy leafy vegetables
- ✓ 1 cup of diced watermelon
- ✓ ¼ cup fresh basil, chopped

Directions:
- ❖ In a small bowl, combine the lemon juice, oil, oregano, thyme, garlic powder and salt. Add the tofu and let it absorb the flavours while you prepare the salad.
- ❖ In a high-speed blender, combine the vinegar and dates and blend until smooth.
- ❖ In each of 4 salad bowls, place 1 cup of leafy greens. Add ¼ cup of watermelon to each.
- ❖ Using a slotted spoon, cover each bowl with 2 tablespoons of vegan feta (store the remaining vegan feta in an airtight container in the fridge for up to 5 days).
- ❖ Garnish evenly with the basil. Pour a spoonful of balsamic mixture over each salad and serve.

34) Spinach and strawberry salad with lemon vinaigrette

Preparation time: 5 minutes   **Cooking time**: 0 minutes   **Portions**: 4

Ingredients:
-   For the lemon vinaigrette
- ✓ 3 tablespoons avocado oil
- ✓ Juice of 1 small lemon
- ✓ 1 teaspoon Dijon or yellow mustard
- ✓ ¼ teaspoon ground turmeric
- ✓ ⅛ teaspoon of sea salt

Ingredients:
- ✓ 1 teaspoon maple syrup (optional)
-   For the salad:
- ✓ 4 cups baby spinach
- ✓ 1 cup of strawberries cut in half
- ✓ ¼ cup sliced almonds

Directions:
- ❖ To make the lemon vinaigrette
- ❖ In a small bowl, whisk together the oil, lemon juice, mustard, turmeric and salt until well combined. Add the maple syrup (if using) and mix well.
- ❖ To make the salad
- ❖ In a large bowl, mix the spinach, strawberries and almonds.
- ❖ Pour the dressing over the salad and toss gently. Serve immediately. Or, if you plan to serve later, store the unseasoned salad and dressing in separate airtight containers in the refrigerator and add the dressing to the salad when you are ready to serve.

35) Rainbow salad with citrus mango dressing

Preparation time: 5 minutes   **Cooking time:** 0 minutes   **Portions:** 4

Ingredients:

For the citrus mango salsa:
- ✓ 2 cups of chopped mango
- ✓ 1 cup chopped fennel
- ✓ ⅓ cup of chopped shallot
- ✓ ¼ cup fresh basil, chopped
- ✓ 3 tablespoons freshly squeezed lemon juice
- ✓ ¼ teaspoon of sea salt

Directions:

- ❖ To make the citrus mango salsa
- ❖ In a medium bowl, combine the mango, fennel, shallot, basil, lemon juice and salt and mix well. For best results, cover and refrigerate for several hours or up to overnight to allow the flavours to meld.

Ingredients:

For the rainbow salad:
- ✓ 1 (15-ounce / 425-g) can low-sodium chickpeas, drained (reserved liquid) and rinsed
- ✓ ½ cup chopped pepper
- ✓ 1 teaspoon chopped fresh coriander, for garnish

- ❖ To make the rainbow salad
- ❖ In a large bowl, combine the chickpeas, pepper and ¼ cup of the sauce. (Store the remaining sauce in an airtight container in the refrigerator for 5-7 days).
- ❖ Garnish the salad with coriander and serve.

36) Roasted cabbage and beetroot salad

Preparation time: 10 minutes   **Cooking time:** 20 minutes   **Portions:** 1-2

Ingredients:

- ✓ 4 small beets, peeled and diced
- ✓ 1 teaspoon avocado oil
- ✓ ¼ teaspoon dried rosemary
- ✓ ⅛ teaspoon of garlic powder
- ✓ Pinch of sea salt
- ✓ Pinch of freshly ground black pepper
- ✓ 2 cups of chopped kale

Directions:

- ❖ Preheat the oven to 400°F (205°C). Line a baking tray with baking paper.
- ❖ In a small bowl, mix the beetroot with the avocado oil to coat. Sprinkle with the rosemary, garlic powder, salt and pepper and toss to coat. Transfer the beets to the prepared baking dish and roast for 15-20 minutes, or until slightly crispy.

Ingredients:

- ✓ ⅛ teaspoon of sea salt
- ✓ 2 tablespoons of avocado oil
- ✓ 1 tablespoon freshly squeezed lemon juice
- ✓ 1 tablespoon brown rice syrup
- ✓ 1 clove of garlic, crushed
- ✓ Pinch of sea salt
- ✓ Pinch of freshly ground black pepper
- ❖ Meanwhile, in a medium bowl, sprinkle the cabbage with the salt, and gently massage the cabbage with your hands, crushing it until soft and slightly mushy, about 3 minutes. Transfer to a serving dish.
- ❖ In a small bowl, whisk together the avocado oil, lemon juice, brown rice syrup, garlic, salt and pepper until well combined.
- ❖ Add the beetroot to the bowl with the cabbage and drizzle with the dressing. Transfer to 1 large or 2 small plates and enjoy.

37) Spelt pasta with avocado

Preparation time: 20 minutes   **Cooking time:** 0 minutes   **Portions:** 4

Ingredients:

- ✓ 4 cups of cooked spelt pasta
- ✓ 1 medium avocado, diced
- ✓ 2 cups of halved cherry tomatoes
- ✓ 1 fresh basil, chopped

Directions:

- ❖ Place the cooked pasta in a large bowl.
- ❖ Add the diced avocado, halved cherry tomatoes and chopped basil to the bowl.
- ❖ Mix all ingredients together until well combined.

Ingredients:

- ✓ 1 teaspoon agave syrup
- ✓ 1 tablespoon lime juice
- ✓ ¼ cup of olive oil

- ❖ Whisk the agave syrup, olive oil, pure sea salt and lime juice in a separate bowl.
- ❖ Pour it over the dough and stir until well combined.
- ❖ Serve immediately.

38) Lettuce and mushroom burger with basil

Preparation time: 15 minutes   **Cooking time**: 20 minutes   **Portions**: 2

Ingredients:

- ✓ 2 cups portobello mushroom caps
- ✓ 1 sliced avocado
- ✓ 1 sliced plum tomato
- ✓ 1 cup of torn lettuce
- ✓ 1 cup of purslane

Directions:

- ❖ Preheat oven to 425°F (220°C).
- ❖ Remove the mushroom stems and cut a ½ inch slice from the top slice, as if slicing a sandwich.
- ❖ Mix the onion powder, cayenne, oregano, olive oil and basil well in a medium bowl.
- ❖ Cover a baking tray with aluminium foil and brush with grapeseed oil to prevent sticking.
- ❖ Place the mushroom caps on a baking tray and brush with the prepared marinade. Marinate for 10 minutes before baking.

Ingredients:

- ✓ ½ teaspoon of cayenne
- ✓ 1 teaspoon of oregano
- ✓ 2 teaspoons of basil
- ✓ 3 tablespoons of olive oil

- ❖ Bake for 10 minutes until golden brown and then turn upside down. Continue baking for a further 10 minutes.
- ❖ Spread the mushroom cap on a serving plate. This will serve as a base for the mushroom burger. On top of it, make a layer of sliced avocado, tomatoes, lettuce and purslane.
- ❖ Cover the burger with another mushroom cap. Repeat steps 7 and 8 with the remaining mushrooms and vegetables.
- ❖ Serve and enjoy.

39) Zoodles with tomato sauce and avocado

Preparation time: 10 minutes   **Cooking time**: 15-20 minutes   **Portions**: 3

Ingredients:

- ✓ 3 medium-sized courgettes
- ✓ 1½ cups of cherry tomatoes
- ✓ 1 avocado
- ✓ 2 sliced green onions
- ✓ ⅓ cup of fresh parsley
- ✓ 1 garlic clove

Directions:

- ❖ Preheat the oven to 400°F (205°C).
- ❖ Cover a baking tray with a piece of baking paper.
- ❖ Place the cherry tomatoes on a covered baking tray. Drizzle with 1 tablespoon of olive oil and season with pure sea salt and cayenne.
- ❖ Cook the tomatoes for about 15-20 minutes until they start to split.
- ❖ Add the avocado quarters, torn parsley leaves, sliced green onions, garlic, spring water, key lime juice and ½ teaspoon pure sea salt to a food processor.

Ingredients:

- ✓ 3 tablespoons of olive oil
- ✓ Juice of 1 key lemon
- ✓ 1 tablespoon of spring water
- ✓ Pure sea salt, to taste
- ✓ Cayenne, to taste

- ❖ Blend until a creamy consistency is achieved. If the sauce is too thick, add more spring water.
- ❖ Cut the ends off the courgettes. Using a spiraliser, make courgette noodles.
- ❖ Mix the courgette noodles with the prepared avocado sauce.
- ❖ Divide between 3 small bowls and serve with cherry tomatoes.
- ❖ Enjoy your zoodles with sauce!

40) Mushroom and pepper fajitas

Preparation time: 10 minutes   **Cooking time**: 10 minutes   **Portions**: 3

Ingredients:

- ✓ 6 tortillas
- ✓ 3 large portobello mushrooms
- ✓ 1 onion
- ✓ 2 peppers
- ✓ 1 teaspoon onion powder

Directions:

- ❖ Rinse the portobello mushrooms and remove the stalks. Cut into ⅓-inch slices.
- ❖ Cut the onion and peppers into thin slices.
- ❖ Add the grapeseed oil to a large frying pan and heat over a medium heat. Add the sliced onions and peppers and cook for 2 minutes.

Ingredients:

- ✓ 1 teaspoon habanero pepper
- ✓ ⅛ teaspoon of cayenne powder
- ✓ Juice of ½ key lime
- ✓ 1 tablespoon grape seed oil

- ❖ Place the sliced mushrooms and seasoning in the pan. Cook for 7-8 minutes, stirring occasionally. Remove from the heat.
- ❖ Take a small frying pan, place the tortillas on it and heat for 30-60 seconds on each side.
- ❖ Place the filling mixture in the centre of the tortillas and pour the lime juice over the vegetables.
- ❖ Serve and enjoy.

41) Chickpea and mushroom sausages

Preparation time: 15 minutes | **Cooking time**: 5 minutes | **Portions**: 8-10

Ingredients:
- ✓ 2 cups of cooked chickpeas
- ✓ 1 quart of Roma tomato
- ✓ 1 cup of quartered mushrooms
- ✓ ½ cup chopped onion
- ✓ ½ cup of chickpea flour
- ✓ 1 tablespoon onion powder
- ✓ 1 teaspoon of ground sage
- ✓ 1 teaspoon of basil

Ingredients:
- ✓ 1 teaspoon of oregano
- ✓ 1 teaspoon of dill
- ✓ ½ teaspoon of ground cloves
- ✓ 1 teaspoon pure sea salt
- ✓ ½ teaspoon of cayenne powder
- ✓ 2 tablespoons of grape seed oil

Directions:
- ❖ Put all the ingredients, except the chickpea flour and grape seed oil, into a food processor.
- ❖ Blend for 15 seconds.
- ❖ Add the chickpea flour to the mixture and blend for a further 30 seconds until well combined.
- ❖ Place the mixture in a piping bag and cut a small piece from the bottom corner.
- ❖ Add the grapeseed oil to a frying pan and heat over high heat.
- ❖ Reduce to a medium heat. Squeeze the prepared mixture into the pan to form sausages.
- ❖ Cook them for about 3 to 4 minutes on all sides. Turn carefully to prevent them from falling apart.
- ❖ Serve and enjoy.

42) Mushroom and kale ravioli

Preparation time: 25 minutes | **Cooking time**: 10 minutes | **Portions**: 5

Ingredients:

Filling:
- ✓ 1 cup of chickpea flour
- ✓ 1 quart of Roma tomato
- ✓ 2 cups of quartered mushrooms
- ✓ 1 cup of chopped cabbage
- ✓ ⅓ cup of diced onions
- ✓ 1 cup diced green and red peppers
- ✓ 1 tablespoon onion powder
- ✓ 1 teaspoon of ginger
- ✓ 2 teaspoons of oregano
- ✓ 2 teaspoons of dill
- ✓ 2 teaspoons of basil
- ✓ 2 teaspoons of thyme
- ✓ 1 teaspoon pure sea salt
- ✓ ½ teaspoon of cayenne

Ingredients:

Dough:
- ✓ ½ cup of chickpea flour
- ✓ 1½ cups of spelt flour
- ✓ ½ teaspoon of oregano
- ✓ ½ teaspoon of basil
- ✓ 1 teaspoon pure sea salt
- ✓ ¾ cup of spring water

Cheese:
- ✓ ½ cup of soaked Brazil nuts (overnight or for at least 3 hours)
- ✓ 2 teaspoons of onion powder
- ✓ ½ teaspoon of oregano
- ✓ 1 teaspoon pure sea salt
- ✓ ½ teaspoon of cayenne powder
- ✓ ½ cup of spring water

Directions:
- ❖ Blend all the filling ingredients, except the chickpea flour, in a food processor for 30-40 seconds.
- ❖ Add the chickpea flour to the mixture and blend until well combined.
- ❖ Add the grapeseed oil to a frying pan and heat over high heat.
- ❖ Reduce to a medium heat. Distribute the ravioli filling in the pan and cook for 3 to 4 minutes on all sides.
- ❖ Break up the filling and cook for a further 3 minutes, then transfer to a medium bowl.
- ❖ Add all the ingredients for the cheese to the food processor and blend until the consistency is creamy. If it is too thick, add a little spring water.
- ❖ Mix the filling with the cheese mixture in the bowl.
- ❖ Place all the dry ingredients for the dough in the food processor and blend for 10-20 seconds. Slowly add the spring water while blending, until the dough can be shaped into a ball.
- ❖ Spread the flour on the work surface. Take ¼ of the dough and roll it out into a thin sheet.
- ❖ Place rounded teaspoons of filling and cheese 1 inch apart on one side of the dough. Fold the dough and press together around the filling to seal. Cut into individual ravioli with a pastry cutter or knife.
- ❖ Repeat steps 9 and 10 with the remaining dough and filling.
- ❖ Bring a pot of spring water to the boil. add a little pure sea salt and grapeseed oil, then cook the ravioli for about 4-6 minutes.
- ❖ Filter and serve.

43) Lettuce wrap and courgette hummus

Preparation time: 10 minutes

Cooking time: 8 minutes

Portions: 2

Ingredients:

- ✓ ½ cup iceberg lettuce
- ✓ 1 courgette, sliced
- ✓ 2 cherry tomatoes, sliced
- ✓ 2 spelt flour tortillas

Directions:

- ❖ Take a grill pan, grease it with oil and preheat it over medium-high heat.
- ❖ Meanwhile, place the courgette slices in a large bowl, sprinkle with salt and cayenne pepper, drizzle with oil and then toss until coated.
- ❖ Place the courgette slices on the grill pan and then cook for 2 to 3 minutes per side until grill marks develop.

Ingredients:

- ✓ 4 tablespoons of homemade hummus
- ✓ ¼ teaspoon of salt
- ✓ ⅛ teaspoon of cayenne pepper
- ✓ 1 tablespoon of grape oil
- ❖ Assemble the tortillas and for this, heat the tortilla on the grill pan until grill marks develop and spread 2 tablespoons of hummus on each tortilla.
- ❖ Spread the grilled courgette slices on the tortillas, cover with lettuce and tomato slices, then wrap tightly.
- ❖ Serve immediately.

44) Apple and pumpkin burger by Butternut

Preparation time: 10 minutes

Cooking time: 1 hour

Portions: 2

Ingredients:

- ✓ ¾ cup diced pumpkin
- ✓ ½ cup diced apples
- ✓ 1 cup cooked wild rice
- ✓ ¼ cup chopped shallots
- ✓ ½ tablespoon of thyme

Directions:

- ❖ Turn on the oven, then set it to 400°F (205°C) and let it preheat.
- ❖ In the meantime, take a biscuit tin, line it with a sheet of parchment, spread the pumpkin pieces on it and then sprinkle with ⅛ teaspoon of salt.
- ❖ Cook the pumpkin for 15 minutes, then add the shallot and apple, sprinkle with the remaining salt and cook for 20-30 minutes until cooked through.
- ❖ When finished, leave the vegetable mixture to cool for 15 minutes, transfer it to a food processor, add the thyme and then pulse until the mixture is chunky.

Ingredients:

- ✓ ¼ teaspoon of sea salt, divided by
- ✓ 1 tablespoon unsalted pumpkin seeds
- ✓ 1 tablespoon of grape oil
- ✓ 2 spelt burgers, halved, toasted

- ❖ Add the pumpkin seeds and cooked wild rice, pulse until combined, then tip the mixture into a bowl.
- ❖ Taste the mixture to adjust it and then shape it into two meatballs.
- ❖ Take a frying pan, place it over a medium heat, add the oil and when it is hot, place the meatballs in it and cook for 5 to 7 minutes per side until golden brown.
- ❖ Place the patties in hamburger buns and then serve.

45) Cabbage and avocado

Preparation time: 5 minutes

Cooking time: 0 minutes

Portions: 2

Ingredients:

- ✓ 1 bundle of cabbage, cut into thin strips
- ✓ 1 small white onion, peeled, chopped
- ✓ 12 cherry tomatoes, chopped

Directions:

- ❖ Take a large bowl, place the cabbage strips in it, sprinkle with salt and then massage for 2 minutes.

Ingredients:

- ✓ 1 tablespoon salt
- ✓ 1 avocado, peeled, stoned, sliced

- ❖ Cover the bowl with plastic wrap or its lid, let it stand for a minimum of 30 minutes, and then stir in the onion and tomatoes until well combined.
- ❖ Let the salad rest for 5 minutes, add the avocado slices and then serve.

46) Courgette bacon

Preparation time: 10 minutes

Cooking time: 20 minutes

Portions: 2

Ingredients:

- ✓ 2 courgettes, cut into strips
- ✓ 1 tablespoon onion powder
- ✓ 1 tablespoon sea salt
- ✓ ½ teaspoon of cayenne powder
- ✓ ¼ cup of date sugar

Directions:

- ❖ Take a medium saucepan, put it over medium heat, add all the ingredients except the courgettes and the oil and then cook until the sugar has dissolved.
- ❖ Then place the courgette strips in a large bowl, pour in the casserole mixture, stir until coated, and then leave to marinate for a minimum of 1 hour.

Ingredients:

- ✓ 2 tablespoons agave syrup
- ✓ 1 teaspoon of liquid smoke
- ✓ ¼ cup of spring water
- ✓ 1 tablespoon of grape oil

- ❖ When you are ready to cook, turn on the oven, set it to 400°F (205°C) and let it preheat.
- ❖ Take a baking tray, line it with a sheet of parchment, grease it with oil, place the marinated courgette strips on top and then bake for 10 minutes.
- ❖ Then turn the courgettes over, continue cooking for 4 minutes and then leave to cool completely.
- ❖ Serve immediately.

47) Mushroom and pepper fritters

Preparation time: 10 minutes

Cooking time: 10 minutes

Portions: 2

Ingredients:

- ✓ 1 cup of chickpea flour
- ✓ 7 ounces (198 g) mushrooms, chopped
- ✓ 1 medium green pepper, core, chopped
- ✓ 1 tablespoon onion powder
- ✓ 2 medium-sized white onions, peeled, chopped
- ✓ 1 teaspoon sea salt

Directions:

- ❖ Take a large bowl, put all the vegetables, add all the seasonings, basil and oregano, mix until combined and then leave the mixture to stand for 5 minutes.
- ❖ Add the chickpea flour, stir until combined and then stir in the water until well combined and smooth.

Ingredients:

- ✓ 1 tablespoon oregano
- ✓ ⅛ teaspoon of cayenne pepper
- ✓ 1 tablespoon of grape oil
- ✓ 1 tablespoon basil leaves, chopped
- ✓ ½ cup of spring water

- ❖ Take a large frying pan, place it over medium heat, add the oil and, when hot, pour the vegetable mixture into portions, press each portion down, and then cook for 3 to 4 minutes per side until cooked and golden brown.
- ❖ Serve immediately.

48) Chickpea, pepper and mushroom curry

Preparation time: 5 minutes

Cooking time: 12 minutes

Portions: 2

Ingredients:

- ✓ 1 cup of cooked chickpeas
- ✓ 1 small white onion, peeled, diced
- ✓ ½ of a medium green pepper, core, chopped
- ✓ 1 cup diced mushrooms

Directions:

- ❖ Take a medium-sized frying pan, place it over medium heat, add the oil and when it is hot, add the onion, tomatoes and pepper and cook for 2 minutes.

Ingredients:

- ✓ 8 cherry tomatoes, chopped
- ✓ ½ teaspoon of salt
- ✓ ¼ teaspoon cayenne pepper
- ✓ 1 teaspoon of grape oil
- ❖ Add the chickpeas and mushrooms, season with and cayenne pepper, stir until combined, and lower the heat to medium-low and then simmer for 10 minutes until cooked through, covering the pan with its lid.
- ❖ Serve immediately.

49) Spelt noodles with peppers and mushrooms

Preparation time: 5 minutes   **Cooking time**: 10 minutes   **Portions**: 2

Ingredients:

- ✓ 2 cups of cooked spelt noodles
- ✓ ½ of a medium green pepper, cored, cut into slices
- ✓ ½ of a medium-sized red pepper, cored, sliced
- ✓ 1 medium white onion, with core, sliced
- ✓ ½ cup of sliced mushrooms

Directions:

- ❖ Take a large frying pan, put it on a medium heat, add the oil and when it is hot, add all the vegetables and cook for 3-5 minutes until tender and crispy.

Ingredients:

- ✓ ⅔ teaspoon of salt
- ✓ ¼ teaspoon of onion powder
- ✓ ⅓ teaspoon of cayenne pepper
- ✓ 1 key lime, squeezed
- ✓ 1 tablespoon sesame oil
- ❖ Add all the spices, sprinkle with the lime juice, stir until combined, then cook for 1 minute.
- ❖ Add the noodles, stir until well mixed and then cook for 2 to 3 minutes until hot.
- ❖ Serve immediately.

50) Okra and tomato curry

Preparation time: 5 minutes   **Cooking time**: 10 minutes   **Portions**: 2

Ingredients:

- ✓ 1½ cups okra
- ✓ 8 cherry tomatoes, chopped
- ✓ 1 medium onion, peeled, sliced
- ✓ ¾ cup of home-made vegetable broth
- ✓ 6 teaspoons of spice mixture

Directions:

- ❖ Take a large frying pan, put it over medium heat, add the oil and heat, add the onion, and then cook for 5 minutes until golden brown.
- ❖ Add the spice mix, add the remaining ingredients to the pan except the okra, stir until combined, and then bring the mixture to a simmer.

Ingredients:

- ✓ ¼ teaspoon of salt
- ✓ ½ tablespoon of grape oil
- ✓ ¼ teaspoon cayenne pepper
- ✓ ¾ cup of tomato sauce, alkaline
- ✓ 6 tablespoons of soft coconut milk jelly
- ❖ Add the okra, stir until combined, and then cook for 10-15 minutes over medium-low heat until cooked through.
- ❖ Serve immediately.

51) Sage mushrooms in the oven

Preparation time: 10 minutes   **Cooking time**: 30 minutes   **Portions**: 2

Ingredients:

- ✓ 2 cups portobello mushrooms, detached
- ✓ ⅔ teaspoon of chopped onion
- ✓ ⅔ teaspoon chopped sage

Directions:

- ❖ Turn on the oven, then set it to 400°F (205°C) and let it preheat.
- ❖ Take an oven dish and then place the mushroom caps in it, cut side up.

Ingredients:

- ✓ ⅔ teaspoon of thyme
- ✓ ⅔ tablespoon of lime juice
- ✓ 2 tablespoons alkaline soy sauce
- ❖ Take a small bowl, put in the remaining ingredients, mix until combined, brush the mixture onto the inside and outside of the mushrooms, and then leave to marinate for 15 minutes.
- ❖ Cook the mushrooms for 30 minutes, turning them halfway through cooking, then serve.

52) Spelt pasta with Swiss chard

Preparation time: 5 minutes   **Cooking time**: 5 minutes   **Portions: 2**

Ingredients:

- ✓ 1 head of Swiss chard, cut into ½ inch pieces
- ✓ 1 cup of spelt pasta, cooked
- ✓ 2 green onions, sliced
- ✓ ¼ cup coriander

Directions:

- ❖ Take a large frying pan, put it over a medium heat, add the oil and when it is hot, add the chard pieces and then cook for 4 minutes or more until they are wilted.

Ingredients:

- ✓ 1 key lime, squeezed, zested
- ✓ ¼ teaspoon of salt
- ✓ ¼ teaspoon cayenne pepper
- ✓ 1 tablespoon olive oil
- ❖ Remove the pan from the heat, transfer the chard to a large bowl, add the remaining ingredients and then stir until combined.
- ❖ Serve immediately.

53) Baked pumpkin and apples

Preparation time: 10 minutes   **Cooking time**: 35 minutes   **Portions: 2**

Ingredients:

- ✓ 1½ pounds (680 g) butternut squash, peeled, seeded and cut into pieces
- ✓ 2 apples, core, cut into ½ inch pieces
- ✓ 2 tablespoons agave syrup

Directions:

- ❖ Turn on the oven, then set it to 375°F (190°C) and let it preheat.
- ❖ Meanwhile, take a baking tray and then spread the pumpkin pieces on it.
- ❖ Take a small bowl, pour in the oil, stir in the salt and allspice until combined, then pour over the pumpkin pieces.
- ❖ Cover the pan with aluminium foil and bake for 20 minutes.

Ingredients:

- ✓ ½ teaspoon of sea salt
- ✓ 2 tablespoons of grape oil

- ❖ Meanwhile, place the apple pieces in a medium bowl, drizzle with the agave syrup and stir until coated.
- ❖ When the pumpkin is cooked, discard the pan, pour the spoonful into the bowl containing the apple and then stir until combined.
- ❖ Spread the apple and pumpkin mixture evenly over the baking tray and then continue baking for 15 minutes.
- ❖ Serve immediately.

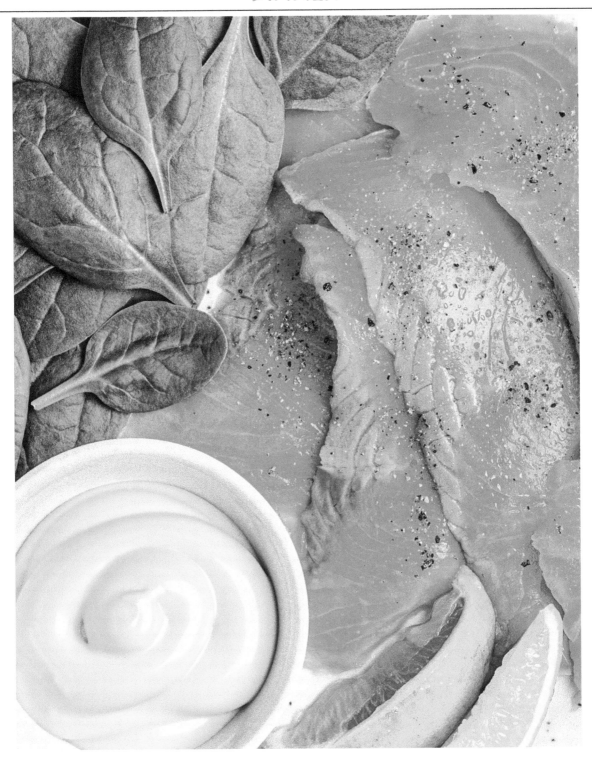

54) Vegetarian stew

Preparation time: 20 minutes   **Cooking time**: 35 minutes   **Portions**: 8

Ingredients:

- ✓ 2 tablespoons of coconut oil
- ✓ 1 large sweet onion, chopped
- ✓ 1 medium parsnip, peeled and chopped
- ✓ 3 tablespoons of homemade tomato paste
- ✓ 2 large cloves of garlic, minced
- ✓ ½ teaspoon ground cinnamon
- ✓ ½ teaspoon ground ginger
- ✓ 1 teaspoon ground cumin
- ✓ ¼ teaspoon cayenne pepper

Ingredients:

- ✓ 2 medium-sized carrots, peeled and chopped
- ✓ 2 medium purple potatoes, peeled and cut into pieces
- ✓ 2 medium sweet potatoes, peeled and cut into pieces
- ✓ 4 cups of homemade vegetable stock
- ✓ 2 cups fresh cabbage, cut and chopped
- ✓ 2 tablespoons fresh lemon juice
- ✓ Sea salt and freshly ground black pepper, to taste

Directions:

- ❖ In a large soup pot, melt the coconut oil over medium-high heat and sauté the onion for about 5 minutes.
- ❖ Add the parsnips and fry for about 3 minutes.
- ❖ Stir in the tomato paste, garlic and spices and fry for about 2 minutes.

- ❖ Stir in the carrots, potatoes, sweet potatoes and stock and bring to the boil.
- ❖ Reduce the heat to medium-low and simmer covered for about 20 minutes.
- ❖ Add the cabbage, lemon juice, salt and black pepper and simmer for about 5 minutes.
- ❖ Serve hot.

55) Quinoa and lentil stew

Preparation time: 15 minutes   **Cooking time:** 30 minutes   **Portions**: 6

Ingredients:

- ✓ 1 tablespoon of coconut oil
- ✓ 3 carrots, peeled and cut into pieces
- ✓ 3 celery stalks, chopped
- ✓ 1 yellow onion, chopped
- ✓ 4 cups of tomatoes, chopped
- ✓ 1 cup of red lentils, rinsed and drained

Ingredients:

- ✓ ½ cup dried quinoa, rinsed and drained
- ✓ 1½ teaspoons of ground cumin
- ✓ 1 teaspoon of red chilli powder
- ✓ 5 cups of vegetable stock
- ✓ 2 cups fresh spinach, chopped
- ✓ Sea salt and freshly ground black pepper, to taste

Directions:

- ❖ In a large frying pan, heat the oil over medium heat and fry the celery, onion and carrot for about 4-5 minutes.
- ❖ Add the garlic and fry for about 1 minute.
- ❖ Add the remaining ingredients except the spinach and bring to the boil.

- ❖ Reduce the heat to low and simmer, covered, for about 20 minutes.
- ❖ Add the spinach and simmer for about 3-4 minutes.
- ❖ Add salt and black pepper and remove from the heat.
- ❖ Serve hot.

292; total fat 6.9 g; saturated fat 1.2 g; cholesterol 0 mg; sodium 842 mg; total carbohydrates 39.1 g; fibre 17.3 g; sugar 6.1 g; protein 19 g

56) Black bean chili

Preparation time: 15 minutes   **Cooking time:**   **Portions**: 6

Ingredients:

- ✓ 2 tablespoons of olive oil
- ✓ 1 onion, chopped
- ✓ 1 small red pepper, seeded and chopped
- ✓ 1 small green pepper, seeded and chopped
- ✓ 4 cloves of garlic, minced
- ✓ 1 teaspoon ground cumin
- ✓ 1 teaspoon cayenne pepper

Ingredients:

- ✓ 1 tablespoon of red chilli powder
- ✓ 1 medium sweet potato, peeled and cut into pieces
- ✓ 3 cups of tomatoes, finely chopped
- ✓ 4 cups of cooked, rinsed and drained black beans
- ✓ 2 cups of homemade vegetable stock
- ✓ Sea salt and freshly ground black pepper, to taste

Directions:

- ❖ In a large frying pan, heat the oil over medium-high heat and fry the onion and peppers for about 3-4 minutes.
- ❖ Add the garlic and spices and fry for about 1 minute.
- ❖ Add the sweet potato and cook for about 4-5 minutes.

- ❖ Add the remaining ingredients and bring to the boil.
- ❖ Reduce the heat to medium-low and simmer covered for about 1½-2 hours.
- ❖ Season with salt and black pepper and remove from the heat.
- ❖ Serve hot.

57) Kidney bean curry

Preparation time: 15 minutes   **Cooking time**: 25 minutes   **Portions: 6**

Ingredients:

- ¼ cup extra virgin olive oil
- 1 medium onion, finely chopped
- 2 cloves of garlic, minced
- 2 tablespoons fresh ginger, chopped
- 1 cup of home-made tomato puree
- 1 teaspoon ground coriander
- 1 teaspoon ground cumin
- ½ teaspoon ground turmeric

Ingredients:

- ¼ teaspoon cayenne pepper
- Sea salt and freshly ground black pepper, to taste
- 2 large plum tomatoes, finely chopped
- 3 cups of boiled red beans
- 2 cups of water
- ½ cup fresh parsley, chopped

Directions:

- In a large soup pot, heat the oil over medium heat and sauté the onion, garlic and ginger for about 4-5 minutes.
- Stir in the tomato puree and spices and cook for about 5 minutes.
- Add the tomatoes, beans and water and bring to the boil over high heat.
- Reduce the heat to medium and simmer for about 10-15 minutes or until the desired thickness.
- Serve hot and garnish with parsley.

58) Green beans in a casserole

Preparation time: 20 minutes   **Cooking time**: 20 minutes   **Portions: 6**

Ingredients:

- For the onion slices:
- ½ cup yellow onion, very thinly sliced
- ¼ cup almond flour
- 1/8 teaspoon of garlic powder
- Sea salt and freshly ground black pepper, to taste
- For the casserole:
- 1 pound fresh green beans, cut up
- 1 tablespoon olive oil

Ingredients:

- 8 ounces fresh cremini mushrooms, sliced
- ½ cup yellow onion, thinly sliced
- 1/8 teaspoon of garlic powder
- Sea salt and freshly ground black pepper, to taste
- 1 teaspoon fresh thyme, chopped
- ½ cup of homemade vegetable stock
- ½ cup of coconut cream

Directions:

- Preheat the oven to 350 degrees F.
- For the onion slices, place all the ingredients in a bowl and mix to coat the onion well.
- Arrange the onion slices on a large baking tray in a single layer and set aside.
- In a pot of boiling salted water, add the green beans and cook for about 5 minutes.
- Drain the green beans and transfer them to a bowl of iced water.
- Drain them well and transfer them again to a large bowl. Set them aside.
- In a large frying pan, heat the oil over medium-high heat and fry the mushrooms, onion, garlic powder, salt and black pepper for about 2-3 minutes.
- Stir in the thyme and stock and cook for about 3-5 minutes or until all the liquid is absorbed.
- Remove from the heat and transfer the mushroom mixture to the bowl with the green beans.
- Add the coconut cream and stir to combine well.
- Transfer the mixture to a 10-inch casserole dish.
- Put the casserole dish and the pan of onion slices in the oven.
- Bake for about 15-17 minutes.
- Remove the tray and foil from the oven and leave to cool for about 5 minutes before serving.
- Cover the casserole dish evenly with the crispy onion slices.
- Cut into 6 equal-sized portions and serve.

59) Vegetarian cake

Preparation time: 20 minutes   **Cooking time**: 20 minutes   **Portions**: 8

Ingredients:

For the gasket:
- ✓ 5 cups of water
- ✓ 1¼ cup of yellow maize flour

For archiving:
- ✓ 1 tablespoon extra virgin olive oil
- ✓ 1 large onion, chopped
- ✓ 1 medium red pepper, seeded and chopped

Ingredients:
- ✓ 2 cloves of garlic, minced
- ✓ 1 teaspoon dried oregano, crushed
- ✓ 2 teaspoons of chilli powder
- ✓ 2 cups fresh tomatoes, chopped
- ✓ 2½ cups cooked pinto beans
- ✓ 2 cups of boiled corn kernels

Directions:

- ❖ Preheat the oven to 375 degrees F. Lightly grease a shallow baking tray.
- ❖ In a pan, add water over medium-high heat and bring to the boil.
- ❖ Slowly add the cornflour, stirring constantly.
- ❖ Reduce the heat to low and cook covered for about 20 minutes, stirring occasionally.
- ❖ Meanwhile, prepare the filling. In a large frying pan, heat the oil over medium heat and fry the onion and pepper for about 3-4 minutes.
- ❖ Add the garlic, oregano and spices and fry for about 1 minute.
- ❖ Add the remaining ingredients and stir to combine.
- ❖ Reduce the heat to low and simmer for about 10-15 minutes, stirring occasionally.
- ❖ Remove from heat.
- ❖ Place half of the cooked cornmeal in the prepared baking tin evenly.
- ❖ Spoon the filling mixture onto the cornflour evenly.
- ❖ Place the remaining cornflour on top of the filling mixture evenly.
- ❖ Bake for 45-50 minutes or until the top is golden brown.
- ❖ Remove the cake from the oven and set aside for about 5 minutes before serving.

60) Rice and lentil meatloaf

Preparation time: 20 minutes   **Cooking time**: 1 hour and 10 minutes   **Portions**: 8

Ingredients:
- ✓ 1¾ cups plus 2 tablespoons of filtered water, divided by
- ✓ ½ cup of wild rice
- ✓ ½ cup of brown lentils
- ✓ Pinch of sea salt
- ✓ ½ teaspoon sodium-free Italian seasoning
- ✓ 1 medium yellow onion, chopped
- ✓ 1 celery stalk, chopped
- ✓ 6 cremini mushrooms, chopped

Ingredients:
- ✓ 4 cloves of garlic, minced
- ✓ ¾ cup rolled oats
- ✓ ½ cup pecans, finely chopped
- ✓ ¾ cup of home-made tomato sauce
- ✓ ½ teaspoon red pepper flakes, crushed
- ✓ 1 teaspoon fresh rosemary, chopped
- ✓ 2 teaspoons fresh thyme, chopped

Directions:

- ❖ In a saucepan, add 1¾ cups of water, the rice, lentils, salt and Italian seasoning and bring to the boil over medium-high heat.
- ❖ Reduce the heat to low and simmer, covered, for about 45 minutes.
- ❖ Remove from the heat and set aside covered for at least 10 minutes.
- ❖ Preheat the oven to 350 degrees F.
- ❖ Using the parchment paper, line a 9x5 inch baking tin.
- ❖ In a frying pan, heat the remaining water over medium heat and fry the onion, celery, mushrooms and garlic for about 4-5 minutes.
- ❖ Remove from the heat and allow to cool slightly.
- ❖ In a large bowl, add the oats, pecans, tomato sauce and fresh herbs and stir until well combined.
- ❖ Add the rice and vegetable mixture to the oat mixture and mix well.
- ❖ In a blender, add the mixture and pulse until it forms a chunky mixture.
- ❖ Transfer the mixture evenly into the prepared baking tin.
- ❖ With a piece of foil, cover the baking tray and bake for about 40 minutes.
- ❖ Uncover and cook for about 15-20 minutes more or until the top is golden brown.
- ❖ Remove from the oven and set aside for about 5-10 minutes before slicing.
- ❖ Cut into slices of the desired size and serve.

61) Asparagus risotto

Preparation time: 15 minutes   **Cooking time**: 45 minutes   **Portions: 4**

Ingredients:
- ✓ 15-20 fresh asparagus spears, trimmed and cut into 1½ inch pieces
- ✓ 2 tablespoons of olive oil
- ✓ 1 cup yellow onion, chopped
- ✓ 1 clove of garlic, chopped
- ✓ 1 cup Arborio rice
- ✓ 1 tablespoon fresh lemon peel, finely grated

Directions:
- ❖ Boil the water in a medium pan then add the asparagus and cook for about 3 minutes.
- ❖ Drain the asparagus and rinse under cold running water.
- ❖ Drain well and set aside.
- ❖ In a large frying pan, heat the oil over medium heat and fry the onion for about 5 minutes.
- ❖ Add the garlic and fry for about 1 minute.
- ❖ Add the rice and fry for about 2 minutes.

Ingredients:
- ✓ 2 tablespoons fresh lemon juice
- ✓ 5½ cups of hot vegetable stock
- ✓ 1 tablespoon fresh parsley, chopped
- ✓ ¼ cup of nutritional yeast
- ✓ Sea salt and freshly ground black pepper, to taste

- ❖ Add the lemon zest, lemon juice and ½ cup of the stock and cook for about 3 minutes or until all the liquid is absorbed, stirring gently.
- ❖ Add 1 cup of stock and cook until all the stock is absorbed.
- ❖ Stirring occasionally, repeat this process, adding ¾ cup of stock at a time until all the stock is absorbed. (This process will take about 20-30 minutes).
- ❖ Stir in the cooked asparagus and the remaining ingredients and cook for about 4 minutes.
- ❖ Serve hot.

62) Quinoa and chickpea salad

Preparation time: 15 minutes   **Cooking time**: 45 minutes   **Portions: 8**

Ingredients:
- ✓ 1¾ cups of home-made vegetable stock
- ✓ 1 cup quinoa, rinsed
- ✓ Sea salt, to taste
- ✓ 1½ cups of cooked chickpeas
- ✓ 1 medium green pepper, seeded and chopped
- ✓ 1 medium red pepper, seeded and chopped

Directions:
- ❖ In a pan, add the stock and bring to the boil over high heat.
- ❖ Add the quinoa and salt and cook again until boiling.
- ❖ Reduce the heat to low and simmer, covered, for about 15-20 minutes or until all the liquid is absorbed.

Ingredients:
- ✓ 2 cucumbers, chopped
- ✓ ½ cup shallots (only the green part), chopped
- ✓ 1 tablespoon olive oil
- ✓ 2 tablespoons fresh coriander leaves, chopped

- ❖ Remove from the heat and set aside covered for about 5-10 minutes.
- ❖ Uncover and stir the quinoa with a fork.
- ❖ In a large serving bowl, add the quinoa and remaining ingredients and stir gently to coat.
- ❖ Serve immediately.

63) Mixed vegetable soup

Preparation time: **Cooking time**:   **Portions:**

Ingredients:
- ✓ 1½ tablespoons of olive oil
- ✓ 4 medium-sized carrots, peeled and chopped
- ✓ 1 medium onion, chopped
- ✓ 2 cloves of garlic, minced
- ✓ 2 stalks of celery, chopped
- ✓ 2 cups fresh tomatoes, finely chopped

Directions:
- ❖ In a large soup pot, heat the oil over medium heat and sauté the carrots, celery and onion for 6 minutes.
- ❖ Add the garlic and fry for about 1 minute.
- ❖ Add the tomatoes and cook for about 2-3 minutes, crushing them with the back of a spoon.

Ingredients:
- ✓ 3 cups of small cauliflower florets
- ✓ 3 cups of small broccoli florets
- ✓ 3 cups frozen peas
- ✓ 8 cups of homemade vegetable stock
- ✓ 3 tablespoons fresh lemon juice
- ✓ Sea salt, to taste
- ❖ Add the vegetables and stock and bring to the boil over a high heat.
- ❖ Reduce heat to a minimum.
- ❖ Cover the pot and simmer for about 30-35 minutes.
- ❖ Add the lemon juice and salt and remove from the heat.
- ❖ Serve hot.

64) Bean and barley soup

Preparation time: 15 minutes   **Cooking time**: 40 minutes   **Portions: 4**

Ingredients:

- ✓ 1 tablespoon olive oil
- ✓ 1 white onion, chopped
- ✓ 2 stalks of celery, chopped
- ✓ 1 large carrot, peeled and chopped
- ✓ 2 tablespoons fresh rosemary, chopped
- ✓ 2 cloves of garlic, minced
- ✓ 4 cups fresh tomatoes, chopped

Directions:

- ❖ In a large soup pot, heat the oil over medium heat and sauté the onion, celery and carrot for about 4-5 minutes.
- ❖ Add the garlic and rosemary and fry for about 1 minute.
- ❖ Add the tomatoes and cook for 3-4 minutes, crushing them with the back of a spoon.

Ingredients:

- ✓ 4 cups of homemade vegetable stock
- ✓ 1 cup pearl barley
- ✓ 2 cups of cooked white beans
- ✓ 2 tablespoons fresh lemon juice
- ✓ 4 tablespoons fresh parsley leaves, chopped

- ❖ Add the barley and stock and bring to the boil.
- ❖ Reduce the heat to low and simmer, covered, for about 20-25 minutes.
- ❖ Add the beans and lemon juice and simmer for another 5 minutes or so.
- ❖ Garnish with parsley and serve hot

65) Tofu and pepper stew

Preparation time: 15 minutes   **Cooking time:** 15 minutes   **Portions:** 6

Ingredients:

- ✓ 2 tablespoons of garlic
- ✓ 1 jalapeño pepper, seeded and chopped
- ✓ 1 (16-ounce) can of roasted red peppers, rinsed, drained and chopped
- ✓ 2 cups of homemade vegetable stock
- ✓ 2 cups of filtered water

Directions:

- ❖ Add the garlic, jalapeño pepper and roasted red pepper to a food processor and pulse until smooth.
- ❖ In a large pan, add the puree, stock and water and cook until boiling over medium-high heat.

Ingredients:

- ✓ 1 medium green pepper, seeded and thinly sliced
- ✓ 1 medium red pepper, seeded and thinly sliced
- ✓ 1 (16-ounce) packet of extra-firm tofu, drained and diced
- ✓ 1 (10-ounce) packet of frozen spinach, thawed

- ❖ Add the peppers and tofu and stir to combine.
- ❖ Reduce the heat to medium and cook for about 5 minutes.
- ❖ Stir in the spinach and cook for about 5 minutes.
- ❖ Serve hot.

66) Chickpea stew

Preparation time: 15 minutes   **Cooking time:** 30 minutes   **Portions:** 4

Ingredients:

- ✓ 1 tablespoon olive oil
- ✓ 1 medium onion, chopped
- ✓ 2 cups carrots, peeled and chopped
- ✓ 2 cloves of garlic, minced
- ✓ 1 teaspoon of red pepper flakes
- ✓ 2 large tomatoes, peeled, seeded and finely chopped

Directions:

- ❖ In a large frying pan, heat the oil over medium heat and fry the onion and carrot for about 6 minutes.
- ❖ Add the garlic and red pepper flakes and fry for about 1 minute.
- ❖ Add the tomatoes and cook for about 2-3 minutes.

Ingredients:

- ✓ 2 cups of homemade vegetable stock
- ✓ 2 cups of cooked chickpeas
- ✓ 2 cups fresh spinach, chopped
- ✓ 1 tablespoon fresh lemon juice
- ✓ Sea salt and freshly ground black pepper, to taste

- ❖ Add the stock and bring to the boil.
- ❖ Reduce the heat to low and simmer for about 10 minutes.
- ❖ Stir in the chickpeas and simmer for about 5 minutes.
- ❖ Add the spinach and simmer for a further 3-4 minutes.
- ❖ Add the lemon juice and the seasoning and remove from the heat.
- ❖ Serve hot.

67) Lentils with cabbage

Preparation time: 15 minutes   **Cooking time**: 20 minutes   **Portions: 6**

Ingredients:
- ✓ 1½ cups of red lentils
- ✓ 1½ cups of home-made vegetable stock
- ✓ 1½ tablespoons of olive oil
- ✓ ½ cup onion, chopped
- ✓ 1 teaspoon fresh ginger, peeled and chopped

Directions:
- ❖ In a pan, add the stock and lentils and bring to the boil over medium-high heat.
- ❖ Reduce the heat to low and simmer, covered, for about 20 minutes or until almost all the liquid is absorbed.
- ❖ Remove from the heat and set aside still covered.

Ingredients:
- ✓ 2 cloves of garlic, minced
- ✓ 1½ cups tomato, chopped
- ✓ 6 cups fresh cabbage, hard ends removed and chopped
- ✓ Sea salt and ground black pepper, to taste

- ❖ Meanwhile, in a large frying pan, heat the oil over medium heat and fry the onion for about 5-6 minutes.
- ❖ Add the ginger and garlic and fry for about 1 minute.
- ❖ Add the tomatoes and cabbage and cook for about 4-5 minutes.
- ❖ Add the lentils, salt and black pepper and remove from the heat.
- ❖ Serve hot.

68) Vegetarian Ratatouille

Preparation time: 20 minutes   **Cooking time**: 45 minutes   **Portions: 4**

Ingredients:
- ✓ 6 ounces of homemade tomato paste
- ✓ 3 tablespoons of olive oil, divided by
- ✓ ½ onion, chopped
- ✓ 3 tablespoons minced garlic
- ✓ Sea salt and freshly ground black pepper, to taste
- ✓ ¾ cup of filtered water
- ✓ 1 courgette, cut into thin circles

Directions:
- ❖ Preheat the oven to 375 degrees F.
- ❖ In a bowl, add the tomato paste, 1 tablespoon of oil, onion, garlic, salt and black pepper and mix well.
- ❖ On the bottom of a 10x10 inch baking tray, spread the tomato paste mixture evenly.

Ingredients:
- ✓ 1 yellow pumpkin, cut into thin circles
- ✓ 1 aubergine, cut into thin circles
- ✓ 1 red pepper, seeded and cut into thin circles
- ✓ 1 yellow pepper, seeded and cut into thin circles
- ✓ 1 tablespoon fresh thyme leaves, chopped
- ✓ 1 tablespoon fresh lemon juice

- ❖ Arrange the vegetable slices alternately, starting at the outer edge of the pan and working concentrically towards the centre.
- ❖ Sprinkle the vegetables with the remaining oil and lemon juice and sprinkle with salt and black pepper and then with thyme.
- ❖ Place a piece of parchment paper on top of the vegetables.
- ❖ Bake for about 45 minutes.
- ❖ Serve hot.

69) Baked beans

Preparation time: 15 minutes   **Cooking time**: 5 hours 5 minutes   **Portions: 4**

Ingredients:
- ✓ ¼ pound of dried lima beans, soaked overnight and drained
- ✓ ¼ pound of dried red beans, soaked overnight and drained
- ✓ 1¼ tablespoons of olive oil
- ✓ 1 small yellow onion, chopped
- ✓ 4 cloves of garlic, minced
- ✓ 1 teaspoon dried thyme, crushed

Directions:
- ❖ Add the beans to a large pot of boiling water and bring back to the boil.
- ❖ Reduce heat to a minimum.
- ❖ Cover the baking tray and bake for about 1 hour.
- ❖ Drain the beans well.
- ❖ Preheat the oven to 325 degrees F.

Ingredients:
- ✓ ½ teaspoon ground cumin
- ✓ ½ teaspoon red pepper flakes, crushed
- ✓ ¼ teaspoon of smoked paprika
- ✓ 1 tablespoon fresh lemon juice
- ✓ 1 cup of homemade tomato sauce
- ✓ 1 cup of homemade vegetable broth
- ❖ In a large oven-proof frying pan, heat the oil over a medium heat and fry the onion for about 4 minutes.
- ❖ Add the garlic, thyme and spices and fry for about 1 minute.
- ❖ Add the cooked beans and other ingredients and immediately remove from the heat.
- ❖ Cover the baking tray and bake in the oven for about 1 hour.
- ❖ Serve hot.

70) Barley Pilaf

Preparation time: 20 minutes   **Cooking time:** 1 hour and 5 minutes   **Portions:** 4

Ingredients:

- ✓ ½ cup pearl barley
- ✓ 1 cup of vegetable stock
- ✓ 2 tablespoons of vegetable oil, divided by
- ✓ 2 cloves of garlic, minced
- ✓ ½ cup white onion, chopped
- ✓ ½ cup green olives, sliced

Directions:

- ❖ In a pan, add the barley and broth over medium-high heat and cook until boiling.
- ❖ Immediately, reduce the heat to low and simmer covered for about 45 minutes or until all the liquid has evaporated.
- ❖ In a large frying pan, heat 1 tablespoon of oil over medium-high heat and fry the garlic for about 30 seconds.
- ❖ Stir in the cooked barley and cook for about 3 minutes.

Ingredients:

- ✓ ½ cup green pepper, seeded and chopped
- ✓ ½ cup of red pepper, seeded and chopped
- ✓ 2 tablespoons fresh coriander, chopped
- ✓ 2 tablespoons fresh mint leaves, chopped
- ✓ 1 tablespoon tamari

- ❖ Remove from heat and set aside.
- ❖ In another pan, heat the remaining oil over medium heat and fry the onion for about 7 minutes.
- ❖ Add the olives and peppers and fry for about 3 minutes.
- ❖ Stir in the remaining ingredients and cook for about 3 minutes.
- ❖ Stir in the barley mixture and cook for about 3 minutes.
- ❖ Serve hot.

71) Vegetable and salmon kebabs

Preparation time: **Cooking time:**   **Portions:**

Ingredients:

- ✓ 4 wooden skewers
- ✓ Pepper (.25 tsp.)
- ✓ Salt (.5 tsp.)
- ✓ Chopped garlic cloves (1)
- ✓ Olive oil (1 tablespoon)
- ✓ Sweet onion cut into quarters (.5)
- ✓ Sliced yellow pepper (1)
- ✓ Cherry Tomatoes (12)
- ✓ Chopped courgettes (1)
- ✓ Salmon (6 oz.)
- ✓ For the plague sauce

Directions:

- ❖ Take out the skewers and thread the vegetables and salmon onto them in the way you prefer.
- ❖ Place them in a baking dish and then brush them with pepper, garlic, salt and olive oil.
- ❖ Turn on the oven and give it time to heat up to 400 degrees. Add the skewers to the oven and bake for a while.

Ingredients:

- ✓ Pepper (.5 tsp.)
- ✓ Salt (1 teaspoon)
- ✓ Olive oil (.25 c.)
- ✓ Pumpkin seeds (.25 c.)
- ✓ Basil leaves (.5 c.)
- ✓ Chopped garlic clove (1)
- ✓ Spinach (1 c.)
- ✓ Lemon juice (1)

- ❖ After 20 minutes, check whether the fish is cooked and then set aside to cool.
- ❖ Take out your blender and put in all the ingredients for the pesto sauce. Add more oil if necessary.
- ❖ Drizzle the pesto sauce over your salmon skewers before serving.

72) Coconut curry with vegetables

Preparation time: **Cooking time:**   **Portions:**

Ingredients:

- ✓ Chopped coriander (3 tbsp)
- ✓ Curry powder (2 teaspoons)
- ✓ Salt (1 teaspoon)
- ✓ Water (.33 c.)
- ✓ Coconut milk (1 c.)
- ✓ Diced tomato (1)
- ✓ Sliced boiled tofu (8 oz)

Directions:

- ❖ Take out a frying pan and heat the coconut oil. When the oil is hot, add the beans, aubergines, peppers, courgettes, ginger and onion.
- ❖ Cook these for five minutes, and then add the tomatoes and tofu. Stir to cook a little longer.

Ingredients:

- ✓ Green beans (.25 lb.)
- ✓ Cubed aubergines (.5 c.)
- ✓ Sliced yellow pepper (1)
- ✓ Diced courgettes (2)
- ✓ Diced yellow onion (.5)
- ✓ Coconut oil (2 tablespoons)

- ❖ After another 5 minutes, add the curry powder, salt, water and coconut milk. Let it simmer for a while.
- ❖ Ten minutes later, the dish is ready. Add the coriander and enjoy!

73) Spaghetti squash loaded

Preparation time: **Cooking time:** **Portions:**

Ingredients:
- ✓ Lemon peel (.5 tsp.)
- ✓ Torn basil leaves (1 c.)
- ✓ Salt (.5 tsp.)
- ✓ Oregano (.5 tsp.)
- ✓ Brown or green lentils, cooked (1 c.)

Directions:
- ❖ Turn on the oven and give it time to heat up to 375 degrees. While it heats up, add a little oil to each spaghetti half and then place them face down on a baking sheet lined with baking paper.
- ❖ Add the pumpkin to the oven and let it cook until tender. After half an hour, the dish should be ready.
- ❖ While this is cooking, heat the rest of the oil in a frying pan. Add the tomatoes, garlic and leaks.

Ingredients:
- ✓ Diced tomatoes (6)
- ✓ Chopped garlic cloves (1)
- ✓ Chopped leek (1)
- ✓ Olive oil (1.5 tablespoons)
- ✓ Spaghetti squash tagliata (1)
- ❖ After eight minutes, you can add the dried oregano and lentils, cooking for another 5 minutes.
- ❖ When the pumpkin is ready, remove it from the oven and use a fork to separate the flesh.
- ❖ Add the lentil and vegetable mixture to this meat and combine.
- ❖ Add the olive oil, lemon zest and torn basil leaves before serving.

74) Spicy pasta

Preparation time: **Cooking time:** **Portions:**

Ingredients:
- ✓ Torn basil leaves (1 c.)
- ✓ Crushed pepper (1 teaspoon)
- ✓ Salt (1 teaspoon)
- ✓ Chilli pepper, diced (1)
- ✓ Sliced black olives (.5 c.)
- ✓ Diced courgettes (.5)
- ✓ Dried tomatoes cut into cubes (.5 c.)

Directions:
- ❖ Use the instructions on the packet to cook the spelt noodles. Drain the water and set aside.
- ❖ Add a little oil to a frying pan before cooking the shallots, carrot, celery and garlic until soft.

Ingredients:
- ✓ Diced cherry tomatoes (2 c.)
- ✓ Diced carrot (1)
- ✓ diced celery stalks (1)
- ✓ Shallots, diced (1)
- ✓ Chopped garlic cloves (1)
- ✓ Olive oil (3 tablespoons)
- ✓ Spelt dough (8 oz)
- ❖ After eight minutes, add the courgettes, sun-dried tomatoes, cherry tomatoes, pepper, salt, chilli and olives.
- ❖ When this is done, throw the pasta into the pan and combine well. Move to a serving dish and cover with a few basil leaves before serving.

75) Stuffed peppers

Preparation time: **Cooking time:** **Portions:**

Ingredients:
- ✓ Peppers, cut tops (2)
- ✓ Crushed pepper (1 teaspoon)
- ✓ Salt (1 teaspoon)
- ✓ Chopped coriander (1 tablespoon)
- ✓ Lime juice (.5)
- ✓ Chilli powder (1 teaspoon)
- ✓ Cumin (1 teaspoon)

Directions:
- ❖ Take out a bowl and combine the avocado, cucumber, diced pepper, lentils and quinoa.
- ❖ In another bowl, whisk together the salt, cilantro, lime juice, chilli, cumin, pepper and olive oil.

Ingredients:
- ✓ Olive oil (2 tablespoons)
- ✓ Diced avocado (.5)
- ✓ Diced cucumber (1)
- ✓ Diced red pepper (1)
- ✓ Cooked green lentils (.5 c.)
- ✓ Cooked quinoa (1 c.)

- ❖ Pour this mixture over the lentil and quinoa mixture and mix. Use this mixture to stuff each pepper before serving.

76) Baba Ganoush Pasta

Preparation time: **Cooking time:**   **Portions:**

Ingredients:
- ✓ Chopped parsley (.25 c.)
- ✓ Cayenne pepper (1 pinch)
- ✓ Salt (.5 tsp.)
- ✓ Vegetable stock (1 tbsp)
- ✓ Chopped chilli pepper (1)
- ✓ Chopped garlic clove (1)
- ✓ Chopped onion (1)

Ingredients:
- ✓ Diced red pepper (.5)
- ✓ Diced courgettes (1)
- ✓ Diced aubergines (1)
- ✓ Olive oil (1 tablespoon)
- ✓ Spelt dough (6 oz)

Directions:
- ❖ Follow the instructions on the packet to cook the spelt pasta and then set it aside.
- ❖ Heat some oil in a frying pan and when the oil is ready, add the chilli, garlic, onion, pepper, courgettes and aubergines to the pan.
- ❖ After 6 minutes of cooking, add the vegetable stock and cook for a further 5 minutes or until hot.

- ❖ Remove it from the oven and leave it to cool for a few minutes before adding it to the blender. Blend until nice and smooth.
- ❖ Add the sauce to your pan and season with a little pepper and salt. Add the cooked pasta and sprinkle with parsley before serving.

77) Broccoli bowl with cheese

Preparation time: **Cooking time:**   **Portions:**

Ingredients:
- ✓ Crushed black pepper (.5 tsp.)
- ✓ Salt (.5 tsp.)
- ✓ Yeast feeding (.24 c.)
- ✓ Lemon juice (1 tablespoon)

Ingredients:
- ✓ Cooked broccoli florets (4 c.)
- ✓ Cooked quinoa (1 c.)
- ✓ Olive oil (1 tablespoon)

Directions:
- ❖ To start this recipe, take out a frying pan and add the oil, broccoli and cooked quinoa.

- ❖ Remove the dish from the heat and serve hot.
- ❖ After five minutes, this should be nice and hot, then add the pepper, salt, nutritional yeast and lemon juice.

78) Green bean and lentil salad

Preparation time: **Cooking time:**   **Portions:**

Ingredients:
- ✓ Shallot (2 tablespoons)
- ✓ Apple cider vinegar (.25 c.)
- ✓ Sliced green beans (2 c.)
- ✓ Halved cherry tomatoes (1 c.)
- ✓ Cooked green lentils (2 c.)
- ✓ Pesto sauce

Ingredients:
- ✓ Salt (1 teaspoon)
- ✓ Olive oil (.25 c.)
- ✓ Chopped garlic clove (1)
- ✓ Pine nuts (2 tablespoons)
- ✓ Spinach (.5 c.)
- ✓ Basil leaves (.75 c.)
- ❖ Pour the pesto sauce over the mixture in the bowl, stir to coat and then serve.

Directions:
- ❖ Take out the food processor and add all the ingredients for the pesto sauce to make it creamy and smooth.
- ❖ In another bowl, combine the vinegar, green beans, tomatoes, lentils and shallots.

79) Vegetable soup

Preparation time:

Cooking time:

Portions:

Ingredients:
- ✓ Spinach (1 c.)
- ✓ Basil (1c)
- ✓ Pepper (1 teaspoon)
- ✓ Salt (2 teaspoons)
- ✓ Oregano (1 tablespoon)
- ✓ Diced tomatoes (1 c.)
- ✓ Vegetable stock (1 tbsp)
- ✓ Kidney beans (.5 c.)

Directions:
- ❖ Take out a stock pot and heat the olive oil in it. When the oil is hot, add the garlic, shallot, carrot, courgette, pumpkin and aubergine to the pot.
- ❖ After five minutes of cooking, add salt, oregano, diced tomatoes, stock, beans and pepper.

Ingredients:
- ✓ Chopped garlic clove (1)
- ✓ Shallot (1)
- ✓ Diced carrot (.5 c.)
- ✓ Diced courgettes (.5 c.)
- ✓ Diced pumpkin (.5 c.)
- ✓ Cubed aubergines (.5 c.)
- ✓ Olive oil (1 tablespoon)

- ❖ Let these ingredients simmer for another ten minutes, adding more spices if desired.
- ❖ Add the spinach and basil just before serving and enjoy.

80) South West Hamburger

Preparation time:

Cooking time:

Portions:

Ingredients:
- ✓ Sliced avocado (1)
- ✓ Lettuce leaves, Bibb (2)
- ✓ Rocket (1c)
- ✓ Dijon mustard (1 tablespoon)
- ✓ Crushed walnuts (1 tablespoon)
- ✓ Nutritional yeast (1 tablespoon)
- ✓ Boiled tofu (4 oz)
- ✓ Crushed black pepper (.5 tsp.)
- ✓ Cayenne pepper (.5 tsp.)

Directions:
- ❖ Heat oil in a frying pan. When the oil is hot, add the onion, pepper, cayenne, cumin, salt, carrot and pepper.
- ❖ After five minutes, the vegetables should be soft. Pour them into a bowl and leave to cool.

Ingredients:
- ✓ Ground cumin (1 teaspoon)
- ✓ Salt (1 teaspoon)
- ✓ Diced carrot (1)
- ✓ Diced green pepper (1 c.)
- ✓ Diced yellow onion (5.)
- ✓ Olive oil (1 tablespoon)

- ❖ Grate the tofu over the bowl and then add the Dijon mustard, walnuts and nutritional yeast. Mix everything together well and form two burgers.
- ❖ Turn on the oven and let it heat up to 400 degrees. Place the burgers on a paper-lined baking tray and then put them in the oven.
- ❖ After half an hour, the burgers should be ready. Remove from the oven and leave to cool before topping with avocado and serving.

81) Courgette rolls with red sauce

Preparation time: **Cooking time:**   **Portions:**

Ingredients:
- ✓ Basil leaves (15)
- ✓ Sliced courgettes (2)
- ✓ Water (.75 c.)
- ✓ Dried oregano (1 teaspoon)
- ✓ Salt (1 teaspoon)
- ✓ Diced red pepper (1)
- ✓ Diced Roma tomatoes (3)
- ✓ Chopped yellow onion (1)
- ✓ Olive oil (1 tablespoon)

Directions:
- ❖ Take out a frying pan and heat some oil in it. Add the oregano, salt, pepper, tomato and onion to make your red vegetable mixture.
- ❖ Cook for a few minutes to make the vegetables soft, and then add a little water. Let it simmer for a while.
- ❖ After ten minutes, remove the pan from the heat and give the vegetable mixture time to cool.
- ❖ Transfer to a blender and blend until smooth.

Ingredients:
- ✓ Basil filling
- ✓ Chopped basil (1 handful)
- ✓ Nutmeg (.25 tsp.)
- ✓ Crushed pepper (.25 tsp.)
- ✓ Salt (.5 tsp.)
- ✓ Nutritional yeast (1 tablespoon)
- ✓ Water (3 tablespoons)
- ✓ Lemon juice (1)
- ✓ Soaked cashews (1 c.)

- ❖ Now, work on the cashew nut filling. Clean the food processor and add all the ingredients until you get a smooth dough. This can take some time, so be patient while doing it.
- ❖ Place the courgette ribbons on a plate in front of you and divide the filling between each one. Roll up each ribbon tightly and then place it in an oven dish with the red vegetable mixture at the bottom.
- ❖ Cover each of these rolls with the rest of the red vegetable mixture and add to the oven which is heated to 375 degrees.
- ❖ After 15 minutes, remove the tray from the oven and leave the dish to cool. Before serving, place the basil leaves on top and enjoy.

82) Meatless Taco Wraps

Preparation time: **Cooking time:**   **Portions:**

Ingredients:
- ✓ Avocado slices (.5)
- ✓ Romaine leaves (4)
- ✓ Water (.25 c.)
- ✓ Salt (.5 tsp.)
- ✓ Cumin (.5 tsp.)
- ✓ Chilli powder (.5 tsp.)
- ✓ Smoked paprika (.5 tsp.)
- ✓ Chopped garlic clove (1)
- ✓ Tomato paste (1 tablespoon)
- ✓ Roasted walnuts (.5 c.)

Directions:
- ❖ Start with the sauce. Add all the ingredients in a bowl and stir to combine. Let marinate for a while while you work on your taco "meat".

Ingredients:
- ✓ Cooked brown lentils (1.5 c.)
- ✓ For the sauce
- ✓ Crushed pepper (.5 tsp.)
- ✓ Salt (.5 tsp.)
- ✓ Apple cider vinegar (1 tablespoon)
- ✓ Chopped coriander (3 tbsp)
- ✓ Diced green pepper (.5 c.)
- ✓ Diced red pepper (.5 c.)
- ✓ Diced mango (.5 c.)

- ❖ Take out the food processor and put together the water, salt, cumin, chilli powder, paprika, garlic, tomato paste, walnuts and lentils. You want this to still be a bit crumbly when you're done.
- ❖ Place the walnut and lentil mixture in each romaine lettuce leaf, and then cover with the sauce and avocado slices before serving.

83) Sesame and quinoa pilaf

Preparation time:

Cooking time:

Portions:

Ingredients:

- ✓ Cooked green lentils (1 c.)
- ✓ Broth or water (1 c.)
- ✓ Quinoa (.5 c.)
- ✓ Chopped garlic clove (1)
- ✓ Diced green pepper (.5 c.)
- ✓ Celery stalk, diced (1)
- ✓ Sliced shallot (1)
- ✓ Crushed pepper (2 teaspoons)
- ✓ Salt (2 teaspoons)
- ✓ Olive oil (2 tablespoons)
- ✓ Sliced carrots (2)

Ingredients:

- ✓ Green beans cut and sliced (1 c.)
- ✓ For the dressing
- ✓ Black sesame seeds (2 tablespoons)
- ✓ Rice vinegar (.25 c.)
- ✓ Tamari (.25 c.)
- ✓ Red pepper flakes (.5 tsp.)
- ✓ Lemon peel (1 teaspoon)
- ✓ Grated ginger (1 teaspoon)
- ✓ Toasted sesame oil (2 tablespoons)
- ✓ Avocado oil (.33 c.)

Directions:

- ❖ Place the carrots and green beans on baking paper on a baking tray. Sprinkle with pepper, salt and a tablespoon of olive oil.
- ❖ Add to the grill of the oven and bake until golden brown. This will take about five minutes.
- ❖ Once this is done, take a pot and add the garlic, pepper, celery, shallot and the rest of the oil.
- ❖ Cook the ingredients for five minutes before adding the quinoa and stirring to cook a little longer.

- ❖ Now add the water or broth and bring to the boil. Let it simmer for a while until the liquid has disappeared.
- ❖ Now you can prepare the dressing. To do this, whisk all the ingredients in a bowl to combine them.
- ❖ When it's time to assemble, mix together the quinoa and lentils. Season with a little pepper and salt and then add the carrot and bean mixture before pouring the dressing over everything.

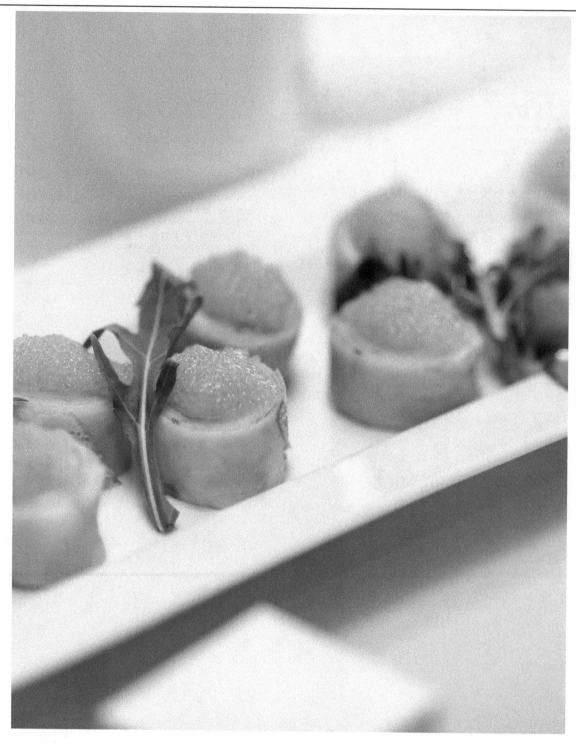

84) Aloo Gobi

Preparation time:

Cooking time:

Servings: 1 bowl

Ingredients:
- ✓ Cauliflower, 750g
- ✓ Fresh ginger, 20g
- ✓ Large onions, 2
- ✓ Mint, 1/3 cup
- ✓ Turmeric, 2 teaspoons
- ✓ Diced tomatoes, 400g
- ✓ Fresh garlic, 2 cloves
- ✓ Cayenne pepper, 2 teaspoons

Ingredients:
- ✓ Cilantro/coriander leaves, 1/3 cup
- ✓ Large potatoes, 4
- ✓ Garam masala, 2 teaspoons
- ✓ Green chilli, 4
- ✓ Water, 3 cups
- ✓ Extra virgin olive oil (cold pressed), 125 ml
- ✓ Salt to taste

Directions:
- ❖ Blend the chilli, garlic and ginger.
- ❖ Fry the oil in a wok for three minutes and add the onion until golden brown.
- ❖ Add the ground pasta and fry for a few seconds, then add; garam masala, chilli, turmeric, tomatoes and salt.

- ❖ Cook for about five minutes and add all the other ingredients.
- ❖ Stir for three minutes and add the water.
- ❖ Cook until the sauce is thick.
- ❖ Serve with Basmati rice or as a side dish.

85) Chocolate Crunch Bars

Preparation time: 3 hours

Cooking time: 5 minutes

Portions: 4

Ingredients:
- ✓ 1 1/2 cups sugar-free chocolate chips
- ✓ 1 cup of nut butter
- ✓ Stevia for taste

Ingredients:
- ✓ 1/4 cup of coconut oil
- ✓ 3 cups pecans, chopped

Directions:
- ❖ Prepare an 8-inch baking tray with baking paper.
- ❖ Mix chips chocolate with butter, coconut oil and sweetener in a bowl.
- ❖ Melt in the microwave for 2 to 3 minutes until melted.

- ❖ Add the cube and nuts. Stir gently.
- ❖ Put this stick in the oven and it will never open again.
- ❖ Refrigerate for 2 to 3 hours.
- ❖ Slice and serve.

86) Walnut butter Bars

Preparation time: 40 minutes.

Cooking time: 10 minutes.

Portions: 6

Ingredients:
- ✓ 3/4 cup of walnut flour
- ✓ 2 ounces of nut butter
- ✓ 1/4 cup Swerve

Ingredients:
- ✓ 1/2 wooden walnut
- ✓ 1/2 teaspoon vanilla

Directions:
- ❖ Combine all the ingredients for a better result.
- ❖ Transfer the contents to a small 6-inch baking tin. Press firmly.

- ❖ Refrigerate for 30 minutes.
- ❖ Cut into slices and serve.

87) Homemade Protein Bar

Preparation time: 5 mnutes

Cooking time: 10 minutes

Portions: 4

Ingredients:
- ✓ 1 knob of butter
- ✓ 4 tbsp. coconut oil
- ✓ 2 scoops of vanilla protein

Ingredients:
- ✓ To taste, ½ tsp of sea salt Optional Ingredients:
- ✓ 1 teaspoon cinnamon

Directions:
- ❖ Mix coconut oil with butter, protein, stevia and salt in a dish.
- ❖ Mix cinnamon and chocolate chips.

- ❖ Presss the dough is firmly and freezed until firmed.
- ❖ Cut the crust into small bars.
- ❖ Serve and enjoy.

88) Shortbread Coookies

Preparation time: 10 minutes   **Cooking time**: 1 hour and 10 minutes   **Portions**: 6

Ingredients:
- ✓ 2 1/2 cups coconut flour
- ✓ 6 tablespoons of nut butter

Directions:
- ❖ Preheat our oven to 350 degrees.
- ❖ Place on a biscuit sheet with the parchment paper.
- ❖ Beat the butter with the erythritol until frothy.
- ❖ Add the vanilla essence and coconut flour.

Ingredients:
- ✓ 1/2 cup erythritol
- ✓ 1 teaspoon of vanilla essence

- ❖ Stir until crumbling.
- ❖ Spoon out a tablespoon of cookie dough onto the cookie sheet.
- ❖ Add more dough to make a pile.
- ❖ Bake for 15 minutes until golden brown.
- ❖ Serve.

89) Coconut biscuits Chip

Preparation time: 10 minutes   **Cooking time**: 15 minutes   **Portions**: 4

Ingredients:
- ✓ 1 cup of walnut flour
- ✓ ½ cup cacao nibs
- ✓ ½ cup coconut flakes, unsweetened
- ✓ 1/3 cup erythritol
- ✓ ½ cup nut butter

Directions:
- ❖ Prepare the oven for 350 degrees F.
- ❖ Layer a cookie sheet with parchment paper.
- ❖ Add and combine all the ingredients dry in a glass bowl.
- ❖ Coconut milk, vanilla, stevia and peanut butter.
- ❖ Beating well stir in the battery. Mix well.

Ingredients:
- ✓ ¼ cup peanut launcher, more than once
- ✓ ¼ cup of coconut milk
- ✓ Stevia, as desired
- ✓ ¼ teaspoon of sea salt

- ❖ Spoon out a tablespoon of cookie dough on the coookie shet.
- ❖ Add more dough to make 16 cooookies.
- ❖ Fluctuate each cookie using your fingers.
- ❖ Water for 25 minutes until dawn.
- ❖ Let them rest for 15 minutes.
- ❖ Serve.

90) Coconut Cookies

Preparation time: 10 mnutes   **Cooking time**: 20 minutes   **Portions**: 6

Ingredients:
- ✓ 6 tablespoons coconut flour
- ✓ ¾ teaspoons baking powder
- ✓ 1/8 teaspoon sea salt
- ✓ 3 tablespoons of nut butter

Directions:
- ❖ Preheat our oven to 375 degrees F. Layer a biscuit sheet with parchment.
- ❖ Place all the wet ingredients in a blender. Blend all the mixture in a blender.
- ❖ Add the wet mixture and mix well until it is absorbed.

Ingredients:
- ✓ 1/6 cup coconut oil
- ✓ 6 tablespoon data sugar
- ✓ 1/3 cup coco nut milk
- ✓ 1/2 teaspoon vanilla essence
- ❖ Place a spoonful of dough cookie on the biscuit sheet.
- ❖ Add a little more butter to make many cooookies. Bake until golden brown (about 10 minutes). We will see.

91) Berry Mousse

Preparation time: 5 minutes   **Cooking time**: 5 minutes   **Portions**: 2

Ingredients:
- ✓ 1 teaspoon Seville orange zest
- ✓ 3 oz. raspberries or blueberries.

Directions:
- ❖ Blend the rice in an electric blender until the fluff is dissolved.
- ❖ Add the vanilla and Seville zest. Stir well.
- ❖ Add the nuts and berries.

Ingredients:
- ✓ ¼ teaspoon vanilla essence
- ✓ 2 cups coconut cream

- ❖ Cover the glove with a plastic key.
- ❖ Refrigerate for 3 hours.
- ❖ Garnish as desired. Serve.

92) Coconut pulp Coookies

Preparation time: 5 minutes.

Cooking time: 10 hours.

Portions: 4

Ingredients:
- ✓ 3 cups coconut pulp
- ✓ 1 Granny Smith apple
- ✓ 1-2 teaspoon cinnamon

Directions:
- ❖ Blend the coconut with the remaining ingredients in a processor food.
- ❖ Make many biscuits with this mixture.
- ❖ Place them on a kitchen table, lined with parchment.

Ingredients:
- ✓ 2-3 tablespoons of raw honey
- ✓ 1/4 cup coco walnut flakes

- ❖ Place the dough in a food oven for 6-10 hours at 115 degrees Fahrenheit.
- ❖ Serve.

93) Avocado Pudding

Preparation time: 10 minutes

Cooking time: 0 minutes

Portions: 2

Ingredients:
- ✓ 2 avocados
- ✓ 3/4-1 cup coconut milk
- ✓ 1/3-1/2 cup of raw cacao powder

Directions:
- ❖ Mix all ingredients in a blender.

Ingredients:
- ✓ 1 teaspoon 100% pure organic vanilla (optional)
- ✓ 2-4 tablespoons of date sugar

- ❖ Refrigerate for 4 hours in a container.
- ❖ Serve.

94) Coconut Raisins cooookies

Preparation time: 10 minutes.

Cooking time: 10 minutes.

Portions: 4

Ingredients:
- ✓ 1 1/4 cups coconut flour 1 cup nut flour
- ✓ 1 teaspoon baking soda
- ✓ 1/2 Celtic teaspoon sea salt
- ✓ 1 peanut button cup
- ✓ 1 cup coconut date sugar

Directions:
- ❖ Turn on the oven to 357 degrees F.
- ❖ Mix the flour with the salt and baking soda.
- ❖ Flatten with sugar until you start and then stirs in walnut milk and vinavilla.

Ingredients:
- ✓ 2 teaspoons of vanilla
- ✓ ¼ cup coconut milk
- ✓ 3/4 cup organic sultanas
- ✓ 3/4 cup coconut chips or flakes

- ❖ Mix well, then place in a container for the powder. Stir until fine.
- ❖ Add all remaining ingredients.
- ❖ Make small coookies out this dough.
- ❖ Place the biscuits on a baking tray.
- ❖ Bake for 10 minutes until set.

95) Cracker Pumpkin Spice

Preparation time: 10 minutes.

Cooking time: 1 hour.

Portions: 6

Ingredients:
- ✓ 1/3 cup coco walnut flour
- ✓ 2 tablespoons pumpkin pie spice
- ✓ ¾ cup sunflower seds
- ✓ ¾ cup flaxseed
- ✓ 1/3 cup sesame seeds

Directions:
- ❖ Heat our oven to 300 degrees F. Combine all ingredients in a bowl.
- ❖ Add the salt and oil to the mixture and mix well.
- ❖ Let the dough rest for 2 to 3 minutes.

Ingredients:
- ✓ 1 tablespoon gron psyllium husk powder
- ✓ 1 teaspoon sea salt
- ✓ 3 tablespoons coco walnut oil, melted
- ✓ 11/3 cups water

- ❖ Roll out the dough on a cookie sheet lined with parchment paper.
- ❖ Bake for 30 minutes.
- ❖ Reduce the amount of food to 30 m and let it rest for another 30 m.
- ❖ Crush the bread into small pieces. Serve

96) Spicy Toasted nuts

Preparation time: 10 minutes.   **Cooking time:** 15 minutes.   **Portions:** 4

Ingredients:

- ✓ 8 ounces of pecans or coconuts or walnuts
- ✓ 1 teaspoon sea salt
- ✓ 1 tablespoon olive oil or coconut oil

Ingredients:

- ✓ 1 teaspoon of ground cumin
- ✓ 1 teaspoon paprika powder or chili powder

Directions:

❖ Add all the ingredients to an oven. Fry the nuts until golden brown.

❖ Serve and enjoy.

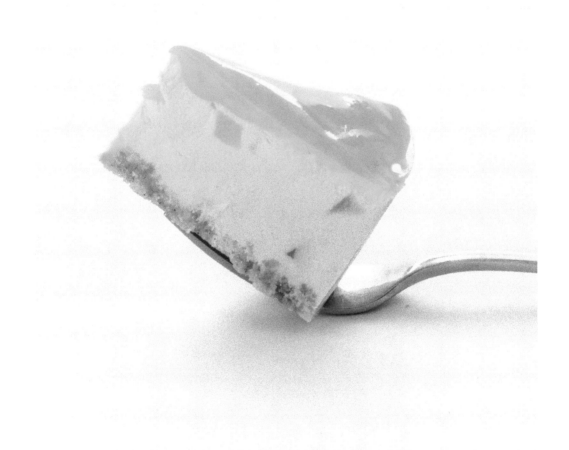

97) Cabbage and pineapple smoothie

Preparation time: 15 minutes   **Cooking time**:   **Portions**: 2

Ingredients:

- ✓ 1½ cups fresh cabbage, chopped and shredded
- ✓ 1 frozen banana, peeled and chopped
- ✓ ½ cup of fresh pineapple chunks

Directions:

- ❖ Add all ingredients to a high-speed blender and pulse until smooth.

Ingredients:

- ✓ 1 cup unsweetened coconut milk
- ✓ ½ cup of fresh orange juice
- ✓ ½ cup of ice
- ❖ Pour the smoothie into two glasses and serve immediately.

98) Green vegetable smoothie

Preparation time: 15 minutes   **Cooking time**:   **Portions**: 2

Ingredients:

- ✓ 1 medium avocado, peeled, pitted and chopped
- ✓ 1 large cucumber, peeled and chopped
- ✓ 2 fresh tomatoes, chopped
- ✓ 1 small green pepper, seeded and chopped

Directions:

- ❖ Add all ingredients to a high-speed blender and pulse until smooth.

Ingredients:

- ✓ 1 cup fresh spinach, torn
- ✓ 2 tablespoons fresh lime juice
- ✓ 2 tablespoons of homemade vegetable stock
- ✓ 1 cup of alkaline water
- ❖ Pour the smoothie into glasses and serve immediately.

99) Avocado and spinach smoothie

Preparation time: 10 minutes   **Cooking time:**   **Portions: 2**

Ingredients:

- ✓ 2 cups of fresh spinach
- ✓ ½ avocado, peeled, pitted and chopped
- ✓ 4-6 drops of liquid stevia

Directions:

- ❖ Add all ingredients to a high-speed blender and pulse until smooth.

Ingredients:

- ✓ ½ teaspoon ground cinnamon
- ✓ 1 tablespoon hemp seeds
- ✓ 2 cups of cooled alkaline water
- ❖ Pour the smoothie into two glasses and serve immediately.

100) Cucumber smoothie

Preparation time: 15 minutes   **Cooking time:**   **Portions: 2**

Ingredients:

- ✓ 1 small cucumber, peeled and chopped
- ✓ 2 cups of fresh mixed vegetables (spinach, cabbage, chard), chopped and shredded
- ✓ ½ cup of lettuce, torn
- ✓ ¼ cup of fresh parsley leaves
- ✓ ¼ cup of fresh mint leaves

Directions:

- ❖ Add all ingredients to a high-speed blender and pulse until smooth.

Ingredients:

- ✓ 2-3 drops of liquid stevia
- ✓ 1 teaspoon fresh lemon juice
- ✓ 1½ cups of filtered water
- ✓ ¼ cup ice cubes

- ❖ Pour the smoothie into two glasses and serve immediately.

101) Apple and ginger smoothie

Preparation time: 10 minutes   **Cooking time:** 0 minutes   **Portions: 1**

Ingredients:

- ✓ 1 apple, peeled and diced
- ✓ ¾ cup (6 oz) of coconut yoghurt

Directions:

- ❖ Add all ingredients to a blender.
- ❖ Blend well until smooth.

Ingredients:

- ✓ ½ teaspoon of freshly grated ginger

- ❖ Refrigerate for 2 to 3 hours.
- ❖ Serve.

102) Blueberry smoothie with green tea

Preparation time: 10 minutes   **Cooking time:** 5 minutes   **Portions: 1**

Ingredients:

- ✓ 3 tablespoons of alkaline water
- ✓ 1 green tea bag
- ✓ 1½ cups of fresh blueberries

Directions:

- ❖ Boil 3 tablespoons of water in a small saucepan and transfer to a cup.
- ❖ Immerse the tea bag in the cup and let it stand for 4 to 5 minutes.
- ❖ Discard the tea bag and
- ❖ Transfer green tea into a blender

Ingredients:

- ✓ 1 pear, peeled, stoned and diced
- ✓ ¾ cup of almond milk

- ❖ Add all other ingredients to the blender.
- ❖ Blend well until smooth.
- ❖ Serve with fresh blueberries.

103)   Apple and almond smoothie

Preparation time: 10 minutes

Cooking time: 0 minutes   **Portions: 1**

Ingredients:

- ✓ 1 cup of apple cider
- ✓ 1/2 cup of coconut yoghurt
- ✓ 4 tablespoons almonds, crushed

Directions:

- ❖ Add all ingredients to a blender.

Ingredients:

- ✓ 1/4 teaspoon of cinnamon
- ✓ 1/4 teaspoon nutmeg
- ✓ 1 cup of ice cubes
- ❖ Blend well until smooth.
- ❖ Serve.

104)   Cranberry smoothie

Preparation time: 10 minutes

Cooking time: 0 minutes   **Portions: 1**

Ingredients:

- ✓ 1 cup cranberries
- ✓ ¾ cup of almond milk
- ✓ ¼ cup raspberries

Directions:

- ❖ Add all ingredients to a blender.

Ingredients:

- ✓ 2 teaspoons fresh ginger, finely grated
- ✓ 2 teaspoons of fresh lemon juice

- ❖ Blend well until smooth.
- ❖ Serve with fresh berries on top.

105)   Berry and cinnamon smoothie

Preparation time: 10 minutes

Cooking time: 0 minutes   **Portions: 1**

Ingredients:

- ✓ 1 cup frozen strawberries
- ✓ 1 cup apple, peeled and diced
- ✓ 2 teaspoons of fresh ginger
- ✓ 3 tablespoons of hemp seeds

Directions:

- ❖ Add all ingredients to a blender.

Ingredients:

- ✓ 1 cup of water
- ✓ ½ lime, squeezed
- ✓ ¼ teaspoon cinnamon powder
- ✓ ⅛ teaspoon of vanilla extract
- ❖ Blend well until smooth.
- ❖ Serve with fresh fruit

106)   Detoxifying berry smoothie

Preparation time: 10 minutes

Cooking time: 0 minutes   **Portions: 1**

Ingredients:

- ✓ 3 peaches, with stone and skin
- ✓ 5 blueberries

Directions:

- ❖ Add all ingredients to a blender.

Ingredients:

- ✓ 5 raspberries
- ✓ 1 cup of alkaline water
- ❖ Blend well until smooth.
- ❖ Serve with fresh kiwi slices.

107) Pink smoothie

Preparation time: 10 minutes

Cooking time: 0 minutes

Portions: 1

Ingredients:

- ✓ 1 peach, core and skin
- ✓ 6 ripe strawberries

Ingredients:

- ✓ 1 cup of almond milk

Directions:

- ❖ Add all ingredients to a blender.
- ❖ Blend well until smooth.
- ❖ Serve with your favourite berries

108) Green apple smoothie

Preparation time: 10 minutes

Cooking time: 0 minutes

Portions: 1

Ingredients:

- ✓ 1 peach, peeled and pitted
- ✓ 1 green apple, peeled and cored

Ingredients:

- ✓ 1 cup of alkaline water

Directions:

- ❖ Add all ingredients to a blender.
- ❖ Blend well until smooth.
- ❖ Serve with apple slices.

AUTHOR BIBLIOGRAPHY

THE ESSENCIAL ALKALINE DIET COOKBOOK FOR BEGINNERS

100+ Alkaline Recipes to Bring Your Body Back to Balance! Healthy Recipes to Enjoy Favorite Foods for Weight-Loss!

THE ALKAINE HEALTHY DIET FOR WOMEN

The Effective Way to Follow an Alkaline Diet comprising Plant-Based Diet Recipes: Natural Ways to Prevent Diabetes! 100+ Recipes Included!

THE ALKAINE HEALTHY DIET FOR MEN

100+ Recipes to Understand pH, Eat Well, and Reclaim Your Health! Plant-Based Recipes Are Included! Boost your Weight-Loss!

THE ALKAINE HEALTHY DIET FOR KIDS

100+ Recipes for Your Health, To Lose Weight Naturally and Bring Your Body Back to Balance

THE ALKALINE FIET COOKBOOK FOR ONE

100+ Recipes to Lose Weight and Get the Benefits of an Alkaline Diet - Alkaline Smoothies Included for Your Way to Vibrant Health - Massive Energy and Natural Weight Loss! Plant-Based Recipes Are Included!

THE ALKAINE DIET FOR WOMEN AFTER 50

2 Books in 1: The Complete Alkaline Diet Guidebook for Beginners: Understand pH, Eat Well with Easy Alkaline Diet Cookbook and more than 200+ Delicious Recipes (Lose weight, Beginners, Foods & Diet, Reset Cleanse)

THE SPECIAL ALKALINE DIET FOR TWO

2 Books in 1: Guidebook for Beginners: Understand pH, Eat Well with Easy Alkaline Diet Cookbook and more than 200 Delicious Recipes! Plant-Based Recipes Are Included!

THE ALKALINE DIET FOR DADDY AND SON

2 Books in 1: For Beginners: The Ultimate Guide of Alkaline Herbal Medicine for permanent weight loss, Understand pH with 200+ Anti Inflammatory Recipes Cookbook! Plant-Based Recipes Are Included!

THE ALKALINE DIET FAST & EASY

2 Books in 1: The Complete and Exhaustive Beginner's Guide to lose Weight, Fasting and Revitalize Your Body with Plant-Based Diet including 200+ Healthy and Tasty Recipes!

THE ALKALINE DIET FOR MUM AND KIDDOS

2 Books in 1: The Simplest Alkaline Diet Guide for Beginners + 200 Easy Recipes: How to Cure Your Body, Lose Weight and Regain Your Life with Easy Alkaline Diet Cookbook! Plant-Based Recipes Are Included!

THE ALKALINE DIET TO LOSE WEIGHT FAST

3 Books in 1: The Revolution of Eating Habits to stay Healthy and Find the Best Shape. A complete Program with 300+ Recipes to Regain a Healthy Balance of the Body with Alkaline Foods and lose Weight Quickly.

THE ALKALINE DIET FOR A HEALTHY FAMILY

3 Books in 1: A Complete Guide for Beginners to Clean and Treat Your Body, Eat Well with More Than 300+ Easy Alkaline Recipes for Weight Loss and Fight Chronic Disease!

THE ALKALINE DIET HIGH-PROTEIN FOR SPORT PLAYERS

3 Books in 1: Diet for Beginners: Top 300+ Alkaline Recipes for Weight Loss with Plant Based Diet And 21 Secrets To Reset And Understand pH Right Now!

THE ALKALINE DIET FOR ABSOLUTE BEGINNERS

3 Books in 1: This Cookbook Includes: Alkaline Diet for Beginners + Alkaline Diet Cookbook, The Best Guidebook to Understanding pH Secrets with More Than 300+ Recipes for Weight Loss and Anti-Inflammatory Action!

THE ALKALINE DIET COMPLETE EDITION FOR EVERYBODY

4 Books in 1: The complete guide to eat well and Lose Weight while understanding pH and prevent disease to boost your everyday energy! 400+ Recipes with Plant-Based Recipes Included!

CONCLUSIONS

Congratulations! You made it to the end!

Thank you for making it to the end of the Alkaline Diet; we hope it was informative and provided all you need to reach your goals, whatever they may be.

With the information you have, you can now start a successful alkaline diet. Your body works best when it's not acidic. The alkaline diet ensures that your body functions at its best. The great thing is that all the food you can eat is tasty. With the recipes in this book, you won't have to worry about making dinner. So don't wait any longer. Start today, and you will see your body change for the better.

The purpose of this cookbook was to introduce readers to most of the insights regarding the alkaline diet in a comprehensive way. Therefore, the text of this book has been categorized into several sections, each of which discusses the basics, the details, what it has and what it doesn't, and recipes related to the alkaline diet. In addition, the recipe chapter is divided into subsections, ranging from breakfast to lunch, dinner, smoothies, snacks, and desserts. So take some time to travel the length of this book and experience the miraculous effects of an alkaline diet on your mind and health.

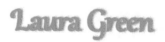

Printed in the USA
CPSIA information can be obtained
at www.ICGtesting.com
LVHW070213260224
772802LV00012B/1027